Positive Options for
Seasonal Affective Disorder (SAD)

Dedication

FOR ALL WHO WOULD LIKE MORE LIGHT
IN THEIR LIVES

Ordering

Trade bookstores in the U.S. and Canada please contact:

Publishers Group West
1700 Fourth Street, Berkeley CA 94710
Phone: (800) 788-3123   Fax: (510) 528-3444

Hunter House books are available at bulk discounts for textbook course adoptions; to qualifying community, health-care, and government organizations; and for special promotions and fund-raising. For details please contact:

Special Sales Department
Hunter House Inc., PO Box 2914, Alameda CA 94501-0914
Phone: (510) 865-5282   Fax: (510) 865-4295
E-mail: sales@hunterhouse.com

Individuals can order our books from most bookstores, by calling **(800) 266-5592**, or from our website at **www.hunterhouse.com**

Positive Options

for

Seasonal Affective Disorder (SAD)

Self-Help and Treatment

Fiona Marshall
and Peter Cheevers

Hunter House Inc., Publishers
PO Box 2914
Alameda CA 94501-0914

Library of Congress Cataloging-in-Publication Data

Marshall, Fiona.
Positive options for seasonal affective disorder (SAD) : self-help and treatment /
Fiona Marshall and Peter Cheevers.
p. cm.
Includes bibliographical references and index.
ISBN 0-89793-414-8 (hbk.) — ISBN 0-89793-413-X (pbk.)
1. Seasonal affective disorder—Popular works. I. Marshall, Fiona. Coping with SAD.
II. Cheevers, Peter. III. Title.
RC545.M37 2003
616.85'27—dc21   2003012852

Project Credits

Cover Design: Brian Dittmar Graphic Design
Book Production: Hunter House
Copy Editor: Kelley Blewster
Proofreader: Rachel E. Bernstein
Indexer: Deanna Butler
Acquisitions Editor: Jeanne Brondino
Editor: Alexandra Mummery
Publicity Coordinator: Lisa E. Lee
Sales & Marketing Coordinator: Jo Anne Retzlaff
Customer Service Manager: Christina Sverdrup
Order Fulfillment: Lakdhon Lama
Administrator: Theresa Nelson
Computer Support: Peter Eichelberger
Publisher: Kiran S. Rana

Printed and Bound by Bang Printing, Brainerd, Minnesota

Manufactured in the United States of America
9 8 7 6 5 4 3 2 1   First Edition   03 04 05 06 07

Contents

Acknowledgments

We are indebted to all the pioneers of light therapy and research into SAD, including Drs. John Ott, Norman Rosenthal, and Jacob Liberman; to all the research done at the National Institute for Mental Health, Washington, D.C.; to research done at the University of Basel, Switzerland; to research done at the University of British Columbia Faculty of Medicine, Vancouver; as well as to work by Professor Chris Thompson and Dr. Ian Rodin at the Royal South Hants Hospital, Southampton, England. We are also indebted to the inspirational work of Primrose Cooper on light and that of Kathleen DesMaisons on nutrition.

Thanks also to all who shared their experiences with us, including Ben Mankowich.

Important Note

The material in this book is intended to provide a review of resources and information related to antiphospholipid syndrome. Every effort has been made to provide accurate and dependable information. However, professionals in the field may have differing opinions, and change is always taking place. Any of the treatments described herein should be undertaken only under the guidance of a licensed health-care practitioner. The author, contributors, editors, publishers, and the experts quoted in the book cannot be held responsible for any error, omission, professional disagreement, outdated material, or adverse outcomes that derive from use of any of the treatments or information resources in this book, either in a program of self-care or under the care of a licensed practitioner.

Introduction

"For the rest of my life I will reflect on what light is," wrote Albert Einstein in 1917. Light is the source of life, and it is also at the very core of our way of life. Whether the source of light be romantic candles or tropical sunshine, the power of light to affect our mood and well-being is tacitly accepted by all of us. It can be no coincidence that light features in so many of our religious festivals, from the Hindu Diwali and the Buddhist Wesak to the Scandinavian Lucia's Day and Jewish Chanukah. It even gives inspiration to the millions of children around the world who celebrate Christmas, which despite its Christian nature is based on ancient pagan celebrations of the return of sunlight after the winter solstice.

Yet many doctors now agree that the past two or three generations of people are the first to spend at least three-quarters of daily life under artificial light. In times gone by, survival dictated that many work outside or near windows during daylight. Over the past few decades, however, those of us who live in the West have been spending more and more of our time indoors. In most cases, we wake indoors, breakfast under artificial light, get into our interior-lit car or train, arrive at our fluorescent-lit office, eat in the subdued light of the lunchroom or restaurant. Even if we manage a lunchtime walk, in many of our major cities tall buildings shade out the light. So for modern-day city dwellers, especially those living in northern latitudes, the sun is seldom seen for large chunks of the year—the exception being the overkill doses we receive on the annual two-week holiday.

The result of our decreased exposure to light is an extraordinary increase in the documentation of SAD, which stands for *seasonal affective disorder*. An estimated one in twenty people suffers from SAD, though it must be remembered that many will fail to notice what they regard as a normal condition of life: feeling low in the winter. Indeed, changes in energy, appetite, mood, and sleep may be observed to some extent in most people during winter. But for those with SAD these symptoms are severe enough to interfere significantly with normal living. In the U.S., an estimated 10 percent of the population suffers from SAD, and this may be a contributing factor to the startling data that one in three people in North America is or has been depressed.

However, there is hope. With the acceptance of SAD as a treatable disorder, people, encouraged by the availability of knowledge in our information age, are beginning to ask questions about the relationship between light and health. They're not just asking how lack of light affects our psychological well-being, but more fundamental, even revolutionary questions. Could there be links between our modern screening out of light and the increase in many diseases? Why are so many degenerative diseases more common in Western societies? Diseases such as hardening of the arteries, senile dementia, multiple sclerosis, and high blood pressure are very common, but is it just diet and lack of exercise that are to blame? Could there be a link between lack of light and these conditions? Could light therapy improve such disorders as hyperactivity, infertility, and respiratory infection?

These ideas go beyond the scope of this book, but the fact that such questions are being looked into suggests that SAD may only be the tip of the iceberg as far as the relationship between light and health is concerned. The effects of sunlight on mood and health— the subject of much research earlier in the last century—remained of marginal medical interest until the 1980s. Since then, serious research has been conducted into SAD. (Research into other conditions has also benefited from the inquiry into light and health. Studies suggest that therapeutic use of light is of benefit in a wide range of settings, including schools and zoos!)

So is the only hope for SAD sufferers to emigrate to a sunnier climate? While a winter holiday may be a great help, light therapy is a highly effective treatment and much more easily available than it used to be. In addition, there are many other ways to help yourself, including diet and exercise. *Positive Options for Seasonal Affective Disorder: Self-Help and Treatment* explores all of these topics. The latest research into SAD suggests that it is the result of an abnormality in the function of serotonin, the hormone that wakes us up and lifts our mood. Serotonin levels are known to fluctuate and to be at their lowest in the winter. Serotonin also influences melatonin, the hormone responsible for making us fall asleep. This book explores the links between SAD, serotonin, and melatonin, and discusses ways to boost serotonin levels.

People have somehow managed to endure SAD for millennia without treatment. However, as *Positive Options for Seasonal Affective Disorder* makes clear, the sufferer of SAD has many choices for improving his or her condition. Seasonal affective disorder can be treated. It is hoped that this book will help sufferers of SAD, as well as their caregivers and families, and be a source of support and reference.

Chapter 1

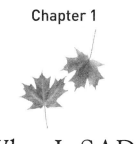

What Is SAD?

"Winter is a disease," wrote the nineteenth-century French poet Alfred de Musset, and many people with seasonal affective disorder (SAD) would wholeheartedly agree with him. Those lowering gray skies seem to invade every corner of your being, flattening all hopes and aspirations and mocking those old summer dreams of happiness. However, this winter disorder can be treated. You can start today, now, and, unless you are very depressed, you may be able to do much of it yourself. Although your doctor may have a part to play in treating SAD, there is a great deal that you can do for yourself to shift the condition, without a huge amount of effort. It can be something as simple as putting down this book, walking over to the window, and taking a long look at the sky. Even on dark days, there will be around ten times more light in the sky than in your room, and absorbing it via your eyes can start to lift your mood (this is explained in more detail later in the book).

Winter depression—also known as "light hunger," "gray-sky syndrome," and "cabin fever"—is not a figment of the imagination, nor is it a new fad. Psychiatrists have known for a long time that mood and emotional disorders can be seasonal. Records exist from 1845 of patients with symptoms that we now know to be indications of SAD, with accompanying doctors' recommendations that the patients winter in sunny Italy instead of Belgium. Later in the nineteenth century, a ship's doctor observed that his crew was becoming increasingly lethargic during the dark days of an Arctic winter; he recommended that their languor be treated with light.

Awareness of seasonal rhythms goes back well before the nineteenth century, however. Hippocrates, in the fifth century B.C., felt that prospective doctors should first get a thorough understanding of seasonal changes and corresponding changes in people and animals. "Some natures are well or ill-adapted for summer, and some for winter. Such diseases as increase in the winter ought to cease in the summer," he wrote. "The doctor too must treat disease with the conviction that each of them is powerful in the body according to the season which is most conformable to it."

Winter is well known for its effects on health. Deaths from all causes peak in January. Hospitalization for depression increases dramatically in the winter months. Family doctors expect to be busier in winter, with an increase in general referrals. This increase is not just due to viral infections, but also to complaints whose causes are sometimes less easy to diagnose—fatigue, sleep problems, and odd aches and pains that may lack a physiological basis. Symptoms like these often indicate SAD.

Despite the condition's long history, the term SAD has only been with us for the past few decades, making it a comparatively recent addition to the list of conditions that can be clinically diagnosed. Yet it is not fully known or understood. SAD often meets with skepticism, from laypeople and the medical profession alike. As one doctor put it, "Who really likes winter?" However, for those going through the misery of SAD, the condition is very real. Many sufferers know they will feel better when the weather changes, and so they just hang on until spring. They often do not seek treatment and therefore are not registered as SAD patients per se. They may find the depression debilitating—and many do—but they manage. Others, however, do not manage. For people with full-blown SAD—about 2 to 3 percent of the population—the disorder can be life-shattering. The serious depression they experience causes them to withdraw from social activities and lose interest in their usual lifestyle. As symptoms worsen with the deepening winter, they may lose their job or an important relationship or drop out of school or college because they can't function. It is vital to take SAD seriously. Indeed, if you think you are suffering from any kind of depression, consult your doctor as soon as possible. Depression is treatable. In any event, if you have any worrisome symptoms, it is worth consulting your doctor before you assume it is SAD. You may be suffering from some other condition, such as chronic fatigue or a viral infection, which can also be treated.

More than the "winter blues," seasonal affective disorder—defined as depression caused by lack of natural light—is now recognized as a condition by the World Health Organization (WHO). However, it is more than just a preference for warm, sunny days over chilly, gray ones. After all, who among us hasn't expressed sentiments such as the following:

I don't mind winter so long as the days are bright; it's those dull cloudy days that get me down.

I always tend to eat more when it's cold.

I can't wait for the spring.

I'm a summer person, definitely.

Many of us undergo seasonal variations in mood, energy, appetite, and sleep between winter and summer. It is not surprising to prefer salads in summer and warming, hearty dishes in winter. It is common to be more energetic and active in spring than in the depths of winter; indeed, much of Western society has organized what amounts to a two-week shutdown in the form of Christmas and New Year's in the darkest part of winter. Many people tend to feel a bit down as the dull winter days wear on and on into January and February, and the first days of real spring sunshine usually bring a general lightening of mood.

The difference with SAD, however, is that sufferers experience an exaggerated version of these mild seasonal blues. In particular, whereas most people cope in spite of these feelings, those with SAD find their ability to function seriously affected—and sometimes disabled. Here is what *Alison*, a thirty-two-year-old teacher, says about SAD:

> Disabling is the word. You are literally less able to carry out normal life—working, driving, seeing friends. Your body goes out of your control because of the bingeing on food that is such a feature of SAD. It's not really about snuggling up early with a hot-water bottle and enjoying it. You feel you're only living half a life because you end up sleeping so much while other people are out there getting on with it. SAD is such an unproductive use of a life—you really feel life is slipping past you while you struggle on, waiting for spring.

This book deals with the best-known form of SAD: a type of winter depression that usually begins as the days shorten, around September or October, and lasts until March or April. In keeping with the shortening days, the condition is often worst between December and February.

SAD has been divided into two levels of intensity:

Sub-SAD or **subsyndromal SAD** affects an estimated 30 percent of all people. It occurs when "normal" winter feelings become more noticeable and begin to affect everyday life. It may overlap with the condition known as "winter vegetative pattern," wherein people's energy levels are lowered but their mood is unaffected.

Full-blown SAD occurs when the depression becomes more disabling, affecting life to the extent that the person finds it difficult to continue with normal activities, such as going out.

In addition, experts have identified different kinds of SAD, each of which can be categorized into the above levels of intensity:

Summer SAD

There's no cure for the summertime blues, it is said. Seasonal variations don't just apply to winter. An estimated 10 percent of seasonal depression takes place in the summer. It may be triggered or intensified by excessive heat and humidity.

Little is known about summer SAD. One of its possible causes may be that some people actually receive less light in hot weather because they spend more time indoors seeking shelter from the sun and/or wear sunglasses when they go out, thus effectively blocking the light from their eyes.

Holiday Blues

SAD is sometimes confused with Christmas depression. Instead of roasting chestnuts by the fire and exchanging gifts in an atmosphere of coziness and warmth, you may be alone and lonely or at bitter loggerheads with the people whom fate has picked out as your family.

The holiday blues can have many causes: sadness that the present can never match up to childhood memories of the event; feelings of being trapped in childhood patterns with parents you have long outgrown; feeling isolated from your usual activities and friends; just feeling isolated; disgust at the commercialism of Christmas; and so on. Such feelings may exist with or without SAD.

Of course, if you do actually have winter depression, you may fail to find Christmas a cheerful day and may continue to be depressed well after the event. If, on the other hand, you do not have SAD, but do suffer from the holiday blues, you probably find that you feel better once the last bits of tinsel have been taken down and you are safely back at work or any other usual routine.

What Causes SAD?

Causes of SAD are looked at in more detail in Chapter 4, but, briefly, besides a lack of light, SAD is thought to be caused by a biochemical imbalance in the brain, featuring a lack of the brain chemical serotonin. In winter, some northern locations only get around eight hours of daylight, as opposed to sixteen hours at the peak of summer. Some individuals with certain brain chemistries seem to be particularly sensitive to this reduction in natural light.

Light, as well as allowing us to see, is used by the body for a variety of metabolic purposes, just as food and water are. Entering the body via the eyes, light stimulates the pineal gland, located in the middle of the brain, to secrete substances that regulate the human biological clock. This in turn influences sleeping, eating, activity levels, and moods—all of which are affected by SAD. In some people, the pineal gland seems to need more outside help in terms of light stimulus in order to function effectively.

Many SAD sufferers come from families in which a parent or close relative suffers from SAD. Indeed, some research suggests that there may be a hereditary factor in at least 30 percent of cases of SAD.

Emotional stress may trigger the depression associated with SAD; on the other hand, there may be no obvious trigger. Everything can be going well in someone's life, but when winter comes, their mood plummets.

SAD symptoms are sometimes explained away by memories of trauma in autumn, especially starting or returning to school. However, the SAD symptoms typically last five or six months—much longer than the initial start of a new school year. Also, and perhaps more importantly, depression from trauma does not usually respond to light treatment, as does SAD.

How Do I Know If It's SAD?

The basic hallmark of SAD is a feeling of overwhelming depression recurring every year during the winter and occasionally during the summer. Symptoms (discussed more fully in Chapter 3) may include extreme tiredness and cravings for carbohydrates, as well as sadness, anxiety, irritability, headaches, weight gain, joint stiffness, lack of interest in sex, and lack of concentration and motivation. Those affected may have difficulty thinking and making decisions or carrying out work and social activities (all symptoms of major depression).

In milder cases, the individual may experience relatively little depression, and may simply feel that his or her energy has dropped.

People usually feel much better in spring and summer, when their mood typically lifts. Around 30 percent of people experience a definite "high" or feeling of elation in spring; for some, this can spill over into mania.

According to the criteria laid down by the WHO, the main symptom to check for is that the depression is seasonal—that is, it starts and ends at particular times of year (usually autumn and spring).

Medical authorities seem to agree that, for a diagnosis of SAD to be made, the following symptoms must be experienced:

◆ the depression lasts for a period of at least 60 days between October/November and March/May;

◆ there must be three episodes, two of which are consecutive;

◆ seasonal depression must outnumber other depressions by three to one;

◆ there should be no environmental factors or stresses, such as being unemployed or isolated from friends in winter.

SAD can be just as severe and serious as other kinds of depression and, like them, if left untreated can wreck the person's quality of life. In extreme cases SAD can even pose a risk of suicide. On the positive side, it is important to remember that depression does pass and that seasonal depression, by its very nature, is likely to lift with the end of winter. Meanwhile, there is a lot that can be done to alleviate the suffering of SAD. This book explores these options in later chapters.

How Common Is SAD?

◆ SAD may affect anyone and begin at any age, but is believed to start mainly between the ages of twenty and forty, with the main sufferers being women in their twenties and thirties.

◆ More women are affected than men; in some areas the proportions are as high as three to one.

◆ SAD has also been documented in children and in the elderly.

◆ SAD has been linked with other conditions, such as PMS (premenstrual syndrome).

◆ Doctors in the U.K. estimate that one in twenty people has been diagnosed with SAD. This figure doesn't take into account those sufferers who have not been diagnosed, of course, so it is possible that this figure is merely the tip of a vast iceberg. According to reports from the National Institute of Mental Health (NIMH) in Bethesda, Maryland, approximately ten million Americans have SAD. If you include sub-SAD, it is estimated that more than thirty million North Americans suffer to some degree from winter depression.

Whereas SAD has been documented throughout the northern and southern hemispheres, it is extremely rare in those living within thirty degrees of the equator, where daylight hours are long, constant, and extremely bright. It is more common in northern latitudes, with people in Scandinavia, Alaska, and Iceland most at risk. The northern parts of the United States and Europe typically have higher rates of alcoholism, depression, family violence, and suicide than places farther south that get more light. In the northern-most parts of the United States, SAD strikes nearly 10 percent of people, as opposed to 1.4 percent in the southern-most states. In Canada, around six hundred thousand people are known to suffer from SAD, according to a survey in Toronto published in the *Canadian Journal of Psychiatry*. It was found that about 3 percent of the Canadian population suffers from seasonal depression—a higher proportion than suffers from other well-researched diseases, such as obsessive-compulsive disorder and schizophrenia.

Alison's Story

Thirty-two-year-old *Alison,* who lived in London, eventually decided to move to Brazil. Here is how she describes her experience of SAD.

I first experienced what I now know to be SAD one autumn in my early twenties. I was working at my first job, I was miles from home and had just ended a relationship, so I had reasons for feeling down and blamed my depression on life events. But, the next autumn, my life situation was much better, and I was surprised when my mood started to plummet again as winter approached with the low gray skies and the endless rain. I kept thinking I should be able to pull myself together and snap out of it, but I couldn't.

That winter, I put on over twenty pounds. I knew I wasn't eating to keep the cold out! I was so tired and unmotivated that I could barely get out of bed. I was frightened of life and of going out and just wanted to put my head under the covers and hide and cry. I didn't realize it at the time, but my thinking was very depressed and morbid—endless thoughts of dying, of time passing. I kept thinking that I was going to die anyway one day, so what was the point of living? It was quite terrifying. I was also very edgy with the kids at school; every little thing seemed to get on my nerves.

This went on for a couple more years. When spring came, I'd be fine—my energy would return, the weight would drop off, and I would be happy and active again. Then, in late autumn, it would all begin again, and I began to blame myself. I felt I was lazy or not organized enough. I was acutely anxious. I felt that life was sliding past me and that I was on the outside, missing out. I didn't have the perspective on my situation to see how my depression was cyclical and varied with the seasons...until I took a winter holiday in the sun.

The difference in how I felt was so striking—and happened so quickly, within a day or two of arriving—that I finally made the connection. Once I had that handle on it, things fell into place quite quickly. My doctor had never heard of SAD, but I researched it myself on the Internet and invested in a lightbox.

Most of my friends thought I was crazy, but when they saw the difference in my moods, they became grudgingly convinced.

Whereas previously I had found it difficult to live a normal life in the winter due to severe depression, suddenly I was again able to go out with my colleagues in the evening for a meal or a concert; I ran a lunchtime and after-school club, and I no longer fell asleep at 8:00 P.M.! The lightbox provided me with just enough light to get me going again. I would still feel a bit down, but it was nowhere near as bad. I made friends with a Brazilian girl, Marta, who also suffered from SAD. I visited her in sunny Brazil and decided to live there for a while and teach English. I know not everyone is in a position to do this, but I think it will be worth it.

Not everyone is so affected by SAD that it makes sense to change countries. However, Alison's story shows what an impact SAD can have on people's lives. Equally important, her tale also demonstrates that SAD can be tackled, and that the experience may even push a person into new ways of living and being that are far more enriching than she or he might have imagined.

Chapter 2

Sunlight Starvation

"There is no area of our mental and bodily functioning that the sun does not influence. We were not designed to hide from it in houses, offices, factories, and schools." So says SAD expert Dr. Damien Downing—and he might have added cars to the list of modern-day structures that keep us out of the sunlight.

Sunlight and good-quality indoor lighting are often overlooked as components of a healthy lifestyle. Yet light is literally life-giving; nothing would exist without it. Light helps the body to produce vitamin D, absorb calcium, and manufacture certain hormones and neurotransmitters that are key to mood and energy level, such as norepinephrine and serotonin. Sunlight is known to trigger a number of biological processes, just like food and water do. Lack of light is the key factor in SAD.

For centuries our work was governed by the amount of daylight available. Although this is still true for farmers and other members of rural communities, in Western industrialized societies we now live indoors, are educated indoors, and work indoors. We spend more time away from the sun than any previous generation did. At the beginning of the twentieth century, more than 70 percent of Americans worked outside. Today, an estimated thirty-eight million North Americans suffer the effects of malillumination (inadequate lighting). Poor lighting creates poor work conditions, which can result in decreased energy and productiveness.

In the U.K., the growth in the number of cases of rickets in the twentieth century was directly linked to lack of daylight caused by crowded buildings and smog in cities, even though the value of sunlight and fresh air in preventing rickets had been noted in 1822. Recently, there has been growing scientific interest in the therapeutic powers of sunlight and of artificial light to treat a wide range of ills, from obesity to cancer. Claims made for the healing power of sunlight go back as far as the ancient Greeks.

How much light do we need? Health experts have suggested that we may have a "minimum daily requirement" of full-spectrum light of between half an hour and two hours. This seems minimal indeed if you consider that our species evolved out-of-doors.

And sunlight is still sunlight even on the cloudiest day. The brightness of light is measured in units called *lux*:

- ◆ 1 lux is equal to the amount of light produced by a single candle;

- ◆ 200 to 700 lux is normal room light indoors;

- ◆ about 100,000 lux is a sunny sky at midday; a cloudy day is around a third of that;

- ◆ around 0.00001 lux—the faintest light—is equal to starlight without the moon shining.

Light treatment for SAD (discussed more fully in Chapter 7) starts at 2,500 lux. This seems to be the minimum amount of light that is required to have a positive effect. New devices for light therapy tend to be more powerful than this. All the same, if you compare lux values indoors with those outdoors, it is easy to see how light starvation happens. Even a cloudy, gray winter's day gives ten times more light than the best-lit office.

Healing Sunlight

Modern humans are believed to have evolved over the past four million years from ancestors who originated in East Africa's Olduvai Gorge, close to the equator. We evolved outdoors, in sunlight.

Anthropologists believe that the human race has spread out from this one location to cover the Earth and has adapted—or has failed to adapt—to the planet's various climates. Could SAD be related to the fact that, as a species, we were designed to live in a sunny climate?

A growing body of scientific opinion supports the idea that our modern lack of both sunlight *and* daylight is damaging our psychological well-being and our general health. Is SAD just the tip of the iceberg?

Because exposure to full-spectrum light has an important influence on the entire human body, some speculate that it can reduce the risks of many diseases, including cancer. No conclusive scientific evidence yet exists for the benefits of "solar therapy," but research certainly suggests that we should all get more daylight and more sunlight—in moderate amounts—and that both kinds of light are extremely helpful for people with SAD.

While using light specifically as an antidepressant is relatively new, heliotherapy—using sunlight to make ourselves feel better—is probably as old as humankind. Light has been used as a medicine for millennia. In the sixth century B.C., Charaka, an Indian physician, treated a number of diseases with sunlight. Hippocrates and other ancient Greek physicians had their patients recuperate in roofless buildings, where they could soak up the rays of the sun.

Too Much of a Good Thing?

The link between excessive exposure to the sun and various skin cancers is well known. In particular, sunburn—especially if you have sensitive skin—has been highlighted as a risk factor for skin cancers. Australia, for example, has the highest rate of skin cancer in the world, long believed to be due to many Australians' prolonged exposure to the sun.

Health-education materials tell us to treat the sun with extreme respect, even fear. This advice is not new. A century ago, colonial Europeans were warned to wear protective "solar topees" (pith helmets) when going out in the African and Asian sun to avoid the dangers of intense sunlight. Sunstroke was an obvious problem, but these fears seem to have had a moral as much as a medical basis. Some doctors believed that the "actinic rays" (that is, rays producing chemical changes) of the sun would sap the vitality of the European stock and lead to degeneration. However, soaking up the hot sun for hours and hours a day year after year is different from getting more daylight during a northern-hemisphere winter. Some influential health practitioners, such as Dr. Jacob Liberman, believe strongly that the dangers of the sun have been greatly exaggerated. While too much strong sunlight (ultraviolet light) may be harmful, a certain amount is necessary to maintain life and health. UV light is said to lower blood pressure, make the heart more efficient, reduce levels of cholesterol, help weight loss, and increase the levels of sex hormones. It also activates the skin hormone solitrol, which works with melatonin (see below). The exact health benefits of the sun are yet to be substantiated by controlled scientific studies, but few people would disagree with the idea that more time spent outside in our technological age can only benefit health.

Advice varies as to how much sunlight is healthy, but, in line with Dr. Damien Downing's advice, the best way to get your sun is in moderation: "in frequent, small doses, insufficient to burn you."

What Sunlight Does to Our Bodies

Light is a key factor in balancing our brain chemicals and hormones so that we go to sleep and wake up appropriately.

When light enters the eye, it hits the cells at the back of the retina (the rods). The nerve signals pass through the optic nerve to the visual cortex of the brain, enabling us to see objects. They also pass to the pineal gland, a pine nut–shaped gland within the hypothalamus that Descartes called "the seat of the soul." Among its many other functions, the pineal gland controls the production of the hormone melatonin, a substance that promotes sleep and, according to some researchers, may even strengthen the immune system.

Your body stops producing melatonin when light reaches an intensity of 2,500 lux. While it closes down the production of melatonin, light also boosts levels of serotonin, making you feel more alert and awake. Toward the end of the day, as the sun goes down and the light disappears, melatonin release begins again with the move toward sleep.

These sleep/wake and dark/light rhythms are part of the body's circadian cycle, a twenty-four-hour biological "clock" that controls the timing of hormone production, body temperature, and other functions besides sleep. This clock is situated within the brain above the eyes, where a small cluster of brain cells (neurons) called the *suprachiasmatic nucleus* (SCN) receives information about the amount of light coming in through the eyes. The light informs the brain how active and alert we need to be, that is, whether it is night and time to rest or day and time to work. Our internal biological clocks are synchronized to the light/dark cycle. In other words, although the body has natural daily rhythms, they are not completely automatic; they rely on cues from light to back them up. The pineal gland seems to act as a kind of radar, scanning the environment to see how much light is present—the major environmental cue.

The pineal gland also influences other areas of the brain, such as the thymus, which is where the T cells that fight infection are produced. That means sunlight is also implicated in the body's immune system; and, indeed, a whole new area of sunlight therapy (based on medical work from the 1920s and 1930s) is emerging.

Sunlight is said to produce a series of metabolic effects in the body that are similar to physical training. For example, tuberculosis patients treated with sunbathing are reported to have well-developed muscles with little or no fat, even though they have not exercised for months. Athletes routinely train in the sun, just as they did in ancient Greece.

Studies suggest that the heart works more efficiently after sunbathing. Sunbathing increases the output of blood from the heart by around 29 percent for five or six days after exposure to ultraviolet light. One study at Tulane University on the effect of sun-light on blood pressure showed that for men with normal blood pressure it had the effect of slightly lowering their blood pressure, an effect that lasted for one or two days. For another group of men in this test who had high blood pressure, sunlight caused an even greater reduction in their blood pressure, an effect that lasted for five or six days.

Conversely, lack of daylight seems to adversely affect the heart. Night-shift workers suffer twice as much heart disease as the rest of us. In some workplaces, night-shift workers are sup-plied with a pair of adjusting glasses or goggles to wear while returning home so that the daylight does not intrude too much into the retina of the eye, which can be uncomfortable for those who are used to the dark. However, use of the goggles, of course, means that the workers are exposed to very little daylight.

Evidence also exists that sunlight lowers cholesterol levels. In one study, rabbits were fed a high-cholesterol diet. Half of the rab-bits were placed in the sun; the others were exposed only to ordi-nary indoor lighting. At the end of the study the sunned rabbits had clean arteries, while the others had severe accumulations and deposits of cholesterol in their arteries.

Evidence shows that exposure to sunlight reduces the risk of developing internal cancers. Research studies in the U.S. and the former U.S.S.R. have shown that breast cancer mortality declines with increasing sunlight intensity. An independent study of prostate cancer in the U.S. showed a similar result, as did a study in 1980 of colon cancer.

Although there is much evidence linking sunlight and malig-nant melanoma, even this connection has been called into ques-tion. Some research has shown that continual exposure to day-light, as with people who work outdoors, actually reduces the risk of melanoma! Some studies find that "intermittent" exposure, as in sunbathing, increases the risk; others do not. Obviously this does not mean that you should cast aside health warnings and rush out to stay in strong sunlight for hours on end. It is a confusing area and one where the "eccentric" element can easily prevail. What does seem clear, however, is that light is certainly linked not just with psychological well-being but with physical health at a profound level. Our attitude to sunlight has been called into question, and the healthy benefits of sunlight or just plain daylight should perhaps be remembered more often in our indoor age.

How It Works

The explanation for the health benefits of sunlight seems to be quite simple. Vitamin D, a hormone, is made (synthesized) in the skin by ultraviolet light. Sunlight is the main source of vitamin D, although it exists in some foods, especially in fortified dairy products and other fortified foods. (The ready availability of fortified foods is the main reason that rickets, a disease of vitamin D deficiency, is almost unheard of anymore in industrialized society, despite the relatively low levels of sunlight we're exposed to.) The role of vitamin D is multifaceted and complex. Besides being essential for bone development, it helps the body absorb calcium.

The twentieth century saw the return of rickets in some areas. It was known as "the English disease" because it was common in crowded, smoggy cities in the U.K. In the U.K., osteoporosis, or fragile bones, presently affects three million women, with one in three at risk. Osteoporosis also has been linked with vitamin D deficiency, especially among older people who may not go outside as much as younger folks and whose ability to synthesize vitamin D declines with age.

Lack of calcium has a number of effects on the body. Whereas 99 percent of the calcium in the body is used by the bones, the remaining 1 percent is vital for:

◆ triggering muscle contractions, including those of the heart;

◆ nerve function;

◆ the activity of several enzymes;

◆ normal blood clotting.

The amount of calcium in the blood is controlled by several hormones, including vitamin D. Vitamin D carries the calcium to and from the bones. Lack of calcium is nearly always due to vitamin D deficiency. (The other cause is extensive surgery on the thyroid gland.)

Lack of vitamin D has been linked with SAD, and it is interesting that joint pain is a symptom of both SAD and vitamin D deficiency. Supplementation, however, is probably not a good idea (see Chapter 10 for details). Vitamin D supplements have not been shown to help people with SAD, according to the small amount of research that has been done. It is definitely unwise to experiment with vitamin D supplementation without supervision by a medical professional, as vitamin D supplements are toxic if taken in excess. Although 400–800 IU daily is a relatively safe dose, excess vitamin D is not easily eliminated from the body. The body's own synthesis, on the other hand, is self-regulating.

It is much easier and safer (and cheaper) simply to get more daylight. Additionally, food sources of vitamin D include cod liver oil and oily fish, such as sardines, herring, mackerel, tuna, salmon, and pilchard. Eggs, liver, and butter provide a little. And most dairy products sold in the U.S. are fortified with vitamin D.

Food sources of calcium include dairy products, such as milk, yogurt, and cheese, canned fish, if you eat the bones, hard water, dried figs, green vegetables, sesame seeds, bread, and flour.

The Effects of Artificial Light

Poor indoor lighting—or "malillumination," to use a term coined by Dr. John Ott—is an accepted feature of many people's indoor environments. Yet it can have a drastic effect, creating symptoms of SAD.

Inadequate artificial lighting at work or school is so common that often we don't even notice it. Conventional fluorescent lights emit light that is deficient in many of the colors and wavelengths of natural sunlight. The usual indoor lighting, which makes use of incandescent bulbs, is mainly a warm yellow or reddish light.

Although this looks cozy, it is deficient in the blue end of the spectrum and contains virtually no ultraviolet light.

Numerous studies have shown the benefits of replacing ordinary fluorescent bulbs with full-spectrum ones, which imitate sunlight more closely. Health at work, health and behavior in prisons, and achievement and behavior at school all improve under full-spectrum lights, as has been shown in large, controlled studies. To discuss all these studies would take more space than is possible here, but let us look at a few. (See "Further Reading," at the back of the book, if you want to explore this subject more.)

The effects of SAD on children's performance at school have been demonstrated by long-term, large studies of schoolchildren. They show that children learn faster in classrooms with good levels of daylight than in darker or artificially lit rooms. One study of schools in Alberta, Canada, found that pupils' performance, especially in verbal creativity, improved greatly when given better light. Students working in rooms that afforded the most natural light had their learning rates improve by 26 percent in reading and 20 percent in math.

In a study at the University of Illinois, sunlight treatments were given to half the members of a physical education class. The experiment ran for ten weeks. At the end of the period, the group that was receiving ultraviolet light had increased their performance on a physical fitness test by almost 20 percent, whereas the other group had improved by just 1 percent. The sunlight-enriched group also suffered half as many colds, their blood pressure went down, and they showed a greater interest in their schoolwork than the sunlight-impoverished group.

Other studies have linked stress, anger, and fatigue at work with the bright glare of fluorescent light, and have shown that natural light has a calming effect, leading to increased energy and productivity. Another study found that sales were 40 percent higher in shops with skylights than in almost identical stores in the same chain that did not have skylights.

Access to natural light is one of the professional standards set for prison authorities. Having enough daylight reduces stress and promotes calm in both inmates and staff and has been shown to reduce levels of violence and further crime. Conversely, there has been concern about links between poor lighting and suicide rates in certain prisons. The first prime minister of India, Nehru, spent a lot of time in prison during India's struggle for independence. A particularly striking passage in his autobiography recalls his suffering from a lack of light in his tiny cell (his only source of light was probably a small kerosene lamp). The image sums up what many sufferers of SAD feel during their winter term of imprisonment. As the Victorian-era poet Emily Dickinson wrote:

> *There's a certain slant of light,*
>
> *On winter afternoons*
>
> *That oppresses…*

The Effects of Light Deprivation

As mentioned, SAD is more common in countries in northern latitudes that receive less light in winter. However, a lack of light can creep up on us in many ways. People who work underground, such as miners, and those who work by night, such as nurses and other shift workers, are obvious examples of people deprived of daylight. But even people working in offices are at risk if the only time they spend in natural light is while walking the few steps from front door to car and from car to entrance. Furthermore, it's not just adults who are deprived of daylight; look at how much time each day the average child spends in a classroom.

Light deprivation can be subtle; you may not even realize you're subject to it. Consider your work environment, which directly influences how much light you get. Your offices might have only a few windows, they may be small, or you might keep the blinds down all the time to prevent glare on your computer screen. The windows may be kept closed or darkened to save energy, or the glass may be coated with light-absorbing substances. Computers themselves, increasingly used, tend to keep people indoors—a factor to be considered with children and teenagers who routinely use the Internet to help with homework or as entertainment. Children also tend to spend more time indoors than past generations because the outside world is perceived as less child-friendly and more dangerous.

Another factor to consider is modern trends in transportation. We walk relatively little and rely on the car much more than our grandparents did, which, again, reduces our exposure to daylight.

The following case histories illustrate how lack of light can cause SAD in people without their suspecting it. It took *Roy* a while to realize what was happening to him.

> Two years ago at the school where I work, an old room was converted into a modern IT (information technology) center, and I was put in charge. It had twenty-two new computers networked to other computers throughout the school and was a source of pride and joy for us all. So enthusiastic was I to get in there and start work that the last thing I noticed was that the room only had three tiny windows near the ceiling. (Previously, the room had been used for storage.)
>
> The new center was ready for use by the start of the academic year. We had a fine, sunny September and October, so all went well. In November, however, I started to feel depressed, which I attributed to problems with a relationship.
>
> By February I started feeling better. The next autumn, though, it was the same story, only worse. In that second year, it was a real struggle to come in to work. I really couldn't understand it. Here I was, with my own little kingdom, and I was desolate. Several times I spent my break feeling close to tears, and sat without speaking to anyone. It all seemed too much. On two occasions I just walked out.
>
> Obviously this could not continue. I was extremely lucky in that I had a sympathetic and informed principal who had been looking at research on the effects of artificial light on schoolchildren. On the second occasion that I walked out, he had a long talk with me in which he mentioned SAD.
>
> Once we realized what was going on, action was taken very quickly. I spent my break, lunch hour, and as much other time as possible out in the open air. I also started light therapy in the

mornings. A larger window was cut into one end of the room. My mood improved dramatically, and I have never looked back. I can hardly believe that the utter misery I went through for two years was simply caused by lack of light.

Moving from a residence that affords a lot of natural light to one that is naturally darker is another cause of depression that is often missed. It is a good idea to view prospective properties on a cloudy day, paying attention to such details as which direction the house faces. Janet's troubles began soon after she moved into a new house.

I had a very pleasant, airy apartment, but because I loved gardening I decided to move out of London to a house and commute in to my job as an administrative assistant. I fell in love with a stone-walled cottage fronted by huge trees.

I loved it in the spring and spent a fantastic summer arranging the garden, inviting friends down for weekends, and generally enjoying life. During autumn, I still spent a fair bit of time in the garden, but when winter came, for the first time I felt really down and lost all my usual energy. I wondered if I had made a mistake moving out of town and found myself making any excuse not to be at home. I'd stay with friends in town during the week or go home to see my parents on weekends.

What I didn't realize was that I had bought an extremely dark, gloomy house. Not only did it face north, but the trees across from it, which were evergreens, effectively blocked all the available light. The trees were privately owned, and the owners refused to have them trimmed. The local town council was unhelpful. I considered converting my attic and putting in lots of skylights, but in the end I reluctantly decided to sell. My first requirement for a new place was its light value. I asked the real-estate agents about window sizes in any property before I even let them send me details about it.

The Climate

Some people's sufferings begin when they move from warmer, southern climes to a more northern latitude with less daylight.

Marta was a Brazilian girl who came to the U.K. to study and work. She thought seasonal depression only happened in people from sunny climates who weren't designed to live in cloudier countries. She was surprised when she met Alison, the English girl whose story is told in Chapter 1.

Changes in weather may also affect some people. Even in summer some find that a few dark, gloomy days or rainy days are enough to set them on the old path of depression. Conversely, in winter, a few fine days may be enough to lift their mood.

Eyeglasses

John Ott—the researcher whose work has aroused interest in SAD—has described how his sunglasses and eyeglasses prevented sunlight from reaching his eyes. Removing them resulted in a drastic improvement in his health. Previously he had suffered from arthritis, frequent colds, and respiratory infections. After breaking his glasses and spending several days in the sun without them, he found that his joints were much easier and looser. A further week in the sun produced even higher levels of fitness.

So it seems that even glasses can be a source of light deprivation; they may prevent light from reaching the pineal gland via the retina. For those interested in finding out more about this subject, Jacob Liberman has written a book titled *Take Off Your Glasses and See* (see "Further Reading," at the back of the book). If you want to try spending time outside without your glasses, it's best to start at times when the sun is not too strong, such as before midmorning or after midafternoon. Never look directly at the sun, even in reduced light, to avoid damaging your eyes.

Another thing to bear in mind is that some people with SAD experience a manic phase in the spring. It is sometimes recommended that they wear dark glasses for part of the day, to calm down the too buoyant effects of the sun.

Chapter 3

The Symptoms of SAD

Is it really SAD you're experiencing, or is it just the winter blues? How do you distinguish SAD from clinical depression? SAD brings with it a number of symptoms, some of which may be confused with those brought on by "ordinary" depression and other disorders. According to the National Institute of Mental Health (NIMH), where pioneering work on SAD was done, and which has researched the subject for more than twenty years, one of the keys to diagnosing SAD is its regularity. It reoccurs from year to year, and always during the same time of year, usually starting around autumn or early winter and lasting until spring.

Here is a summary of the main factors that set SAD apart from clinical depression and other disorders:

- ◆ **seasonal depression**—starting and ending at a certain time of the year, usually in autumn and spring, respectively, and characterized by feelings of hopelessness, guilt, misery, anxiety, and sometimes by suicidal thoughts

- ◆ **increased desire to sleep**—oversleeping, difficulty waking up in the morning, and daytime drowsiness

- ◆ **extreme fatigue and lethargy**—lack of energy and motivation; feeling too tired to perform ordinary tasks

◆ **increased appetite and craving for simple carbohydrates and sweets,** often leading to weight gain

However, SAD can be as idiosyncratic as any other condition and may well include other symptoms, as you will see from the checklist and case histories included in this chapter. An individual's experience of SAD may also differ from year to year, with slightly different symptoms or with some years being more severe than others. According to the NIMH, although people with SAD may not experience severe symptoms every year, around seven out of ten winters are very difficult for them.

As touched on in Chapter 1, besides overt SAD, there is a less severe, subclinical seasonal pattern known as the "winter blues," familiar to many people. Dr. Norman Rosenthal, the physician who named and defined SAD, speaks of a "gray zone" between the blues and SAD. According to Rosenthal, who has worked extensively with the NIMH and is now clinical professor of psychiatry at Georgetown University, many individuals who suffer from the winter blues mistakenly diagnose themselves as having SAD. They may have less energy or be less productive or creative, but fail to experience the sleep problems that characterize clinical cases of SAD. It is when the condition becomes disabling that there is cause for concern.

If you feel you may be suffering from depression, it is important that you consult your doctor as soon as possible. He or she can help. Review the list of SAD symptoms below, which includes many signs of depression. In particular, symptoms may include negative thinking that is hard to shake off, difficulty finishing tasks you previously found quite manageable, and persistent thoughts of death. Furthermore, SAD symptoms can mimic other serious medical conditions, such as thyroid problems or chronic fatigue, and these also need medical attention, so it is wise to check with your doctor before undertaking a plan of self-care.

SAD Symptoms: A Checklist

At some time in their lives, many people experience some of the feelings and behaviors listed below. Many of these symptoms can indicate other forms of depression. Bear in mind that the first six in particular distinguish SAD from other conditions. Some research suggests that SAD symptoms may become worse in the late afternoon, as dusk falls. This is another factor to consider when monitoring your feelings.

1. Depression that starts and stops suddenly at regular times of the year

2. Eating more than usual

3. Craving carbohydrates and sweets

4. Weight gain as a result of satisfying these cravings

5. Extreme tiredness

6. Sleeping more than usual

7. Lack of energy and loss of interest in activities

8. Sleep disturbance

9. Feelings of sadness and hopelessness

10. Cognitive problems; difficulty concentrating and making decisions. Tasks you previously found simple now seem complicated

11. Drinking more alcohol than usual

12. Drinking more coffee and tea than usual

13. Anxiety, tension, and low tolerance of stress

14. Phobias

15. Irritability

16. Social withdrawal

17. Blaming others or circumstances

18. Wanting to stay at home rather than go out

19. Loss of libido

20. Menstrual problems. Premenstrual tension may be worse than usual, with attendant irritability, sleep problems, appetite changes, and low energy levels

21. Low body temperature

22. Minor physical ailments, such as increased sensitivity to pain, headaches, muscle and joint pain; digestive problems such as irritable bowel, constipation, diarrhea; palpitations and night sweats

23. More prone to infections such as colds and flu

24. Keener sense of smell, and changes in taste

Symptoms in Children and Teenagers

Chapter 4 covers the topic of SAD in children and teens in greater detail, but the list of symptoms below is a useful starting point. The following signs are probably typical of all children at some time, especially toward the end of a hard week at school. However, if they are unusually pronounced or occur only in autumn or winter, they may indicate SAD. Symptoms to look out for include

1. Irritability

2. Bad behavior

3. Tantrums and crying

4. Reduced performance at school

5. Loss of interest in usual activities, especially sports

6. Depression

7. Not wanting to see friends

8. Sleep problems at night, and sleepiness by day

9. Unusual craving for junk foods and sweets

10. Reluctance to do jobs around the house that he or she usually does not mind doing

11. Headaches and other minor disorders

Case Histories

The following real-life experiences illustrate how SAD can affect people. *Sally,* a forty-one-year-old mother, felt that she simply couldn't cope with the combined demands of her job and family.

> I had terrible mood swings and felt very low and depressed. I was also very tired all the time—unnaturally so. My memory was terrible; I'd go to a store and forget what I went in for. I know everyone does this, but it was slowing my day down noticeably. I got nothing done. I felt that I was being unfair to the children and ruining their lives. At the same time, I became really snappy and irritated with them, screaming and shouting all the time. They seemed so badly behaved.
>
> When my husband came home from work, I would complain that the children went to him and didn't want me. Of course they wanted him because they hadn't seen him all day. I was quite irrational. I remember standing in the kitchen thinking, "If I go to my doctor and say I'm depressed, they may take the children away." This seemed a very real possibility. I felt I was losing my mind.

Marie, a thirty-three-year-old lab technician, said she went into "hibernation mode."

> It's as if your whole system slows down. You don't want to go out, you don't want to have people around, you just want to be left alone. It's an effort to go to the store and too much bother sometimes to take a bath—easier just to crawl back into bed. Sometimes I didn't even bother to change from my day clothes into pajamas and just spent days in the same clothes. The only thing I was interested in was sweets. I developed a passion for them, all kinds, and would spend ages deciding whether I was going to have chocolate or hard candies and where I was going to get them.

Jon, a thirty-nine-year-old counselor, suffered a range of "horrible" symptoms.

> A lot of my symptoms were physical. I had lots of aches and pains, to the point where I was taking paracetamol (acetaminophen) all the time. I had digestive problems, including terrible gas! Night sweats were a real problem; I'd wake up drenched. And total fatigue—I just want to lie down all the time. I had an absolute craving for sun and sunshine and always felt better if we took a winter vacation. I forgot things all the time—PIN numbers, phone numbers. I lost interest in food and sex.

Atypically, Jon ate less and even lost weight in winter—around six or seven pounds. Also unusually for a SAD sufferer, he slept less and woke up very early—a classic symptom, in fact, of clinical depression. However, he knew he was suffering from SAD, first because it came on so suddenly around the middle of September, and second because it was cured by light therapy. Nevertheless, it is worth pointing out again that SAD and clinical depression can overlap, and both can be treated.

Both Sally and Jon had suffered seasonal depression all of their adult lives. Jon remembered having it in his twenties, and Sally recalled experiencing periods of depression as a child (SAD in children is discussed more fully in Chapter 4).

The next few sections examine some of the prominent SAD symptoms in more detail.

Depression

Depression is the key factor in SAD, with mood being so drastically changed as to affect most aspects of life. Feelings of sorrow or grief, a loss of self-esteem, hopelessness, and even despair are all typical. Many people find it hard to work; statistics show that time taken off work by SAD sufferers increases dramatically in winter.

Depression can show itself in different ways. For example, some people feel guilty, perhaps for their lack of energy or for overeating. Irritability is another symptom, sometimes leading to feelings of violence. As with clinical depression, you may feel you want to withdraw from the world and avoid social contact. These are feelings we may all experience at times, but in SAD sufferers they may persist and affect many aspects of normal behavior, including relationships.

Depression can also be masked as anxiety, panic, loss of confidence, and paranoid thoughts. Poor memory and concentration are common. SAD can literally make a different person of you.

Barry, who was in his mid-twenties, experienced depression severe enough that he was admitted to the same hospital year after year, usually in late September and generally for several months. Every year around February, he became better and was able to go home within a few days of his mysterious recovery. The nurses first noticed that he acted more sociable. Then he began to pay more attention to personal hygiene, changing his clothes and bathing again. One day they heard music coming from his room and only then discovered that he was a talented musician and had hidden his flute under his bed. Through all the winters he had been hospitalized, no one had known until that day that he even owned a flute! The nurses had known only the "droopy" patient who would barely do a thing for himself; yet here was an energetic young musician who seemed a completely different person.

Increased Desire to Sleep

The need for extra sleep can be disabling in severe cases of SAD. Sleep disturbance is a classic symptom of clinical depression; in such cases it usually manifests as early waking or inability to sleep. By contrast, the urge to sleep longer is characteristic of SAD. At the SAD clinic at the Royal South Hants Hospital, in Southampton, U.K., a study of two hundred SAD sufferers showed that they needed two and a half to three hours more sleep each night in winter than in summer.

SAD patients may find themselves falling asleep earlier in the evening, or may have difficulty getting out of bed in the morning. Although sufferers may be sleeping longer than usual, they may still feel tired or drowsy during the day. Again, from *Alison:*

I felt I could not get enough sleep. I resented being woken, no matter what the time, but I didn't realize that I had already slept more than enough until my partner pointed it out to me. He became quite irritated at first, at having a hibernating bear slumbering away all evening and all night. Then he became concerned, saying that ten hours a night was what a growing child needed, not an adult. In fact, it was the sleeping that first made me go to the doctor. My partner became worried that it was a sign of some illness, such as narcolepsy, and made me go. Needless to say I came back after various blood tests for anemia and so on with a clean bill of health and not much the wiser; my doctor thought I had "maybe had a virus recently."

Some SAD sufferers wake up during the night, or their sleep may be restless and less satisfying—two possible causes for fatigue. Equally, the fatigue may persist even when a person has slept a solid eight to ten hours, and some individuals may show signs of sleep deprivation, such as irritability and foggy thinking. These symptoms may be linked to low levels of brain chemicals. Current thinking on SAD points to a brain-chemical imbalance as a prime factor in the disorder (this is explained more fully in Chapter 4).

Extreme Lethargy

One survey has shown that the extreme tiredness or lethargy that sufferers feel is what they find most disturbing about SAD. It may take different forms, including an inability to concentrate at work, a loss of interest in usual activities, or a general lack of vitality, as experienced by *Patrick:*

It's just as if you were hibernating during the cold, dark months. I'd procrastinate about work and put as much as I could on hold. I couldn't make decisions. Facts would go round and round in my head, and I lost the ability to organize them or to edit them. I was usually pretty good at throwing away junk mail and other trash the minute it hit my desk. With SAD, that ability seemed to go out of the window. I literally couldn't bring myself to look through all the reams of paper I seemed to receive—I just didn't have the energy. I kept my office door closed and my head low. Some days I'd just give up and go home. I felt "too tired" the whole time, and close to tears. Some days I could have wept at work, and on a few I did. Those were generally the days I went home early.

Increased Appetite and Weight Gain

As if to combat the lack of energy, many people crave particular foods and may eat more than usual, sometimes bingeing. Indeed, SAD has been linked with eating disorders, such as bulimia and anorexia. The main foods people seem to crave are simple carbohydrates and starchy foods: pasta, white bread, cakes, cookies, sweets.

The overeating can cause weight gain ranging from around seven to thirty pounds. In the study at the SAD clinic at the Royal South Hants Hospital, 69 percent of those taking part reported increased appetite, and 73 percent craved high-energy foods. They reported a tendency to avoid salads and healthy foods, and they all gained weight. Again, eating a bit more and gaining a few pounds is a normal occurrence during winter, but not usually to this extreme.

It is common for those with SAD to feel as if they have no control over their excessive eating. Some believe that the urge to eat more simple carbohydrates may be a form of self-medication, an instinctive attempt to raise levels of the neurotransmitter (brain messenger chemical) serotonin, which influences mood. The way this works is explained more fully in Chapter 8, but it is useful to note here that this theory also explains why many patients respond favorably to selective serotonin-reuptake inhibitors (SSRIs) and antidepressants such as Prozac or Zoloft.

In spring and summer, eating habits usually return to normal, and people tend to lose the extra weight they have gained in winter—only to regain it the following winter. This cyclical problem is compounded by the fact that sometimes not all the weight is lost, with the result that some SAD sufferers end up overweight or even obese in the long term. This subject is tackled in Chapter 8, where we take a look at the theory that carbohydrate cravings are triggered by a lack of the brain chemical serotonin.

Comfort Drinking

Some individuals find that they drink more caffeinated beverages and/or alcohol during winter.

The caffeine in coffee, tea, and sodas can be a powerful draw for people who are trying to combat the lethargy they feel. Caffeine dilates the pupils in the eyes, allowing in more light, which can boost serotonin production. For this reason, increased coffee drinking can be seen as an instinctive attempt at self-medication for SAD. According to research from St. Elizabeth's Medical Center, in Boston, there is also evidence that coffee can mimic the effect of light in birds, and may help to shut down melatonin production in humans. This is possibly another attempt by the body to treat itself.

Some symptoms resulting from excessive caffeine intake can mimic those of depression. These include indigestion, stomach pains, nervousness, panic attacks, palpitations, and sleep problems.

Alcohol may also be used as a quick comfort. Because it provides the body with a simple sugar, it boosts certain brain chemicals and blood-sugar levels temporarily, raising the sufferer's mood for a while. Again, alcohol cravings are thought to be a sign of decreased levels of serotonin. On the psychological side, for those who don't feel like getting their usual exercise, an evening spent at a bar can be an easy way to fill time on a winter's night.

Too much alcohol can, of course, cause a wide range of symptoms, both physical and emotional, from headache to remorse. The long-term effects of consuming excessive quantities of alcohol are well known and include damage to the liver, heart, and brain cells. Furthermore, alcohol is a natural depressant, so once the immediate effects have worn off, the drinker with SAD tends to feel lower than before.

Seasonal Mood Swings

One feature of SAD is the way the sufferer's mood lifts in the spring. Many people feel an increase in energy and a dramatic improvement in mood. As if to make up for lost time, some throw themselves into work, tackling and completing projects with a surge of enthusiasm.

For some people with SAD—though not all—this "spring fever" can spill over into a manic phase (hypomania), which brings problems of its own. Ordinary judgment and the instinct for self-preservation seem to be blunted. Sufferers may find that they need far less sleep and rest and charge around expending energy without allowing adequate time to recharge their batteries. They may spend too much money and be generally impulsive, perhaps starting new relationships or jobs on the spur of the moment, upsetting old arrangements, and disrupting relationships generally.

Although they have a lot of energy, it tends to be very unfocused. Because they are easily distracted, they may have loads of ideas for projects that they start but fail to finish. A disregard for personal safety may spill over into aspects of daily life, such as driving, where greater recklessness brings an increased risk of accidents. *Patrick* had a revelation about this:

> I would have a difficult month in April. I would speed through every aspect of my life. I'd walk faster, work more quickly, and talk faster. My wife taped me talking during a manic phase. It was instructive! I literally talked much faster than normal and flitted about from subject to subject, and woe to anyone who tried to interrupt me. It was as if I had lost the ability to listen. I was also very argumentative, usually about trivial things. By May I would have calmed down.

As stated, "spring fever" does not affect every SAD patient. Some simply resume a normal productive life with feelings of relief, while others endure a stormier course through spring and may suffer ups and downs in line with the unpredictable weather.

Recognizing SAD

A classic symptom of depression is failing to realize that you have it! SAD is no exception.

Steve, a thirty-two-year-old banker, suffered several puzzling symptoms each winter and felt awful, but he didn't know why. He lost interest in his usual activities, felt very tired and unmotivated, was tearful and irritable, and experienced sleep problems. He was much more emotionally sensitive than normal and felt he had less staying power to endure the trials of everyday life.

I couldn't believe this was happening to me each winter. It went on for years until, one day, sitting in the office, I picked up a phrase on the Internet that led me to an article on SAD. It was a revelation. As I read, I could tick off almost word for word the list of symptoms. The article informed me that what I was feeling was the norm for SAD. I could have shouted with relief.

Sally didn't realize just how depressed she was.

It's really difficult to see that it is depression when you're in the middle of it. I would have gone on like that if one day a friend hadn't dropped by. I told her I just wanted to walk out and leave everyone behind. She said, "This isn't like you." She made me go to my doctor and even sat with the children during my appointment. My doctor prescribed antidepressants, which were wonderful. My friend also suggested that we meet up in the mornings and go to the park with our children. Now that I know more about SAD, I understand that the daylight helps as much as getting out and having a break from the home routine.

Again, both these stories underline how important it is to go to your doctor or to talk to a friend you trust. Don't suffer in silence.

SAD and Suicide

People tend to talk about seasonal depression in an ironic tone. It can be seen as a bit of a whimsical disorder. People who've never encountered it in themselves or in someone they know may wonder if it really exists. Nevertheless, it is important to bear in mind that in extreme cases SAD is not only very real but can be life threatening. As with other forms of depression, the risk of suicide should be taken seriously—the more so because SAD is preventable, with treatment.

At the Sleep Disorders Center in an American psychiatric hospital, a thirty-five-year-old woman with SAD was admitted as an emergency patient after trying to commit suicide and nearly succeeding. The doctor who talked to her found out that she suffered from SAD every winter, but was usually able to hang on until her children's spring break in February, when the family went to sunny Florida. The vacation immediately lifted her spirits. This year, the February holiday hadn't come until the first week of March. She had been unable to bear it any longer.

SAD Is Treatable

Although awareness of SAD has been heightened over the past decade, many still live in darkness, both metaphorically and literally, with regard to the disorder. Millions of people who have varying degrees of SAD grit their teeth and just live through their symptoms for yet another winter, not realizing that, like other forms of depression, it is a treatable condition. The woman whose near tragic story is described above was successfully treated with bright light. (This treatment is explained more fully in Chapter 7.)

Many assume that they are simply not winter people. They don't pursue treatment because they know their condition will likely improve with the arrival of spring. Why suffer, though, when you can do something about it? The remedies are covered in Chapters 5 to 10.

Chapter 4

Serotonin and
Other Factors

The latest research suggests that SAD is linked with an abnormality in the way serotonin functions. The brain chemical serotonin, or 5HT, is a neurotransmitter (nerve messenger) controlled by the hypothalamus, which is the part of the brain that controls mood, appetite, sleep, and sex. Enough serotonin makes people feel calm, centered, and balanced, while a lack of it is a well-known factor in clinical depression.

In SAD, serotonin's role is implicated with that of melatonin, the hormone that induces sleep. It's a bit like a seesaw: too little serotonin results in too much melatonin, which is thought to be one reason for SAD sufferers' feelings of lethargy and lack of energy. The extra melatonin primes the body for sleep, doing so all day long rather than after nightfall, as is normal. Overcoming SAD is believed to be a matter of getting this brain chemistry back in balance. Chapters 5 to 10 look at ways to do this, including light therapy, diet, and exercise.

Light deprivation is regarded as the main cause of SAD, but with our increased understanding of the brain, it might be more accurate to instead call it the main *trigger*. Whereas some people seem inherently more vulnerable to SAD—perhaps because of genetic factors—they may never develop it. Lack of light seems to be the factor that tips the vulnerable into actual depression. This can happen in various and sometimes unexpected ways, as we saw in Chapter 2 with the stories of Janet, who moved to a darker house, and Roy, who had to work in a room without natural light. Other theories exist about what causes SAD. Some speculate that it may be linked with abnormalities in bilirubin, a substance in the blood. However, at this time there is no way of making artificial bilirubin, so treatment using bilirubin remains only a possibility for the future. This chapter focuses on factors that can be dealt with, such as serotonin levels. Furthermore, as with any depression or mood disorder, life stresses may contribute to SAD, although sufferers usually agree that winter is the main trigger. *Rachel* voices a common finding:

> Tasks that I sail through in the summer are so much harder, sometimes impossible, in winter. In other words, my life can be going fine, but as the dull, dark days close in, every little thing seems too much.

Dr. Norman Rosenthal, who identified SAD, believes that it may have more than one cause, or may have different causes in different people, with serotonin imbalances being responsible in some cases, melatonin in others, and both in yet others. As with other forms of depression, individual variations have to be taken into account.

The Serotonin Factor

Interestingly, levels of serotonin are seasonal and are at their lowest in the winter. Good levels of serotonin are likely to make you feel balanced, optimistic, and in control. Serotonin is a neurotransmitter—that is, a chemical messenger within the nervous system. It carries signals inside the brain, allowing the hypothalamus to "speak" to the area of the brain that controls sleep/wake cycles, the *substantia nigra*. If this communication process is impaired, then disturbances of mood and sleep tend to result. Besides making you feel depressed, lower levels of serotonin may also make you feel scattered and unfocused in your thinking, impair your ability to concentrate easily, and give you a short attention span. You may find work frustrating or be unable to complete a project that you know is well within your grasp.

Serotonin also influences impulse control. Impulse control enables you to refuse temptations such as those glazed doughnuts brought to the office by a coworker, a double mocha latte, or an extra glass of wine. Lack of serotonin, therefore, may lead to impulsive actions, such as eating a chocolate bar or flying into a rage, simply because your brain is not giving you enough time to think decisions through before acting.

Research has linked low levels of serotonin not only with depression but also with an increased craving for simple carbohydrates, such as pasta, bread, cakes, and sweets. This craving is believed to be the brain's response to low levels of serotonin; eating more starchy, sugary foods is an instinctive attempt to boost levels of serotonin in the brain. Unfortunately, the effect is only temporary. Chapter 8 looks at how the right diet can boost serotonin levels naturally.

Levels of serotonin can be raised by taking the drug Prozac or a similar SSRI (selective serotonin-reuptake inhibitor). Research has also linked exposure to bright light with the increased production of serotonin.

As mentioned previously, serotonin influences the production of melatonin, which leads us to the next part of the story.

Melatonin: Nature's Sedative

Melatonin is a hormone that helps control when we sleep and wake up. Identified in 1958, it has since been found to regulate many other hormones involved in controlling our circadian rhythm—that is, our twenty-four-hour pattern of sleep and wakefulness. Melatonin also controls reproductive hormones in women, thereby affecting menstrual cycles and menopause. Disturbances in melatonin production could be one reason why SAD is more common in women. Melatonin also indirectly causes body temperature to drop, which may be another factor contributing to loss of energy and depression. Children have the highest levels of melatonin. The body's levels drop with age, which perhaps explains why older people tend to sleep less or to suffer sleep disturbances. Like serotonin, levels of melatonin fluctuate with the seasons. They are at their lowest during spring and summer because melatonin can only be produced in quantity during hours of darkness, which are relatively fewer in the warm seasons. Conversely, the fewer the hours of daily light in winter, the longer is the period of time during which melatonin can be produced. Thus, it will have a stronger effect at that time of year, making you feel more lethargic.

Normally, daytime levels of melatonin are very low and undetectable. Melatonin is excreted in high concentrations via the urine each morning, as shown in a study on morning auto-urine drinking (drinking one's own morning urine is a traditional practice within yogic religion and is still widely performed to help achieve meditative states). In people with SAD who do this, daytime levels of melatonin tend to be higher.

Some research has also linked higher daytime levels of melatonin with an increase in the craving for carbohydrates. Because carbohydrates create energy and raise body temperature, higher melatonin levels could result in the need for more carbohydrates to help create more energy and body warmth.

Dopamine

Dopamine is another brain chemical that is present in the retina. Its production is stimulated by light and suppressed by melatonin. Again, abnormalities in dopamine production and suppression are thought to be linked with SAD.

Genetic Factors

Is heredity a causal factor in SAD? It can be. Many SAD sufferers come from a family where a parent or close relative suffers from SAD. One study that looked at SAD in pairs of twins found that where one twin had the disorder, about half of the other twins also had it. Other work has shown that there is a hereditary factor in at least 30 percent of cases.

Researchers have discovered a gene that may make people more vulnerable to SAD. For a long time it was suspected that SAD had a genetic component since it tends to run in families. Indeed, around 70 percent of sufferers have one relative who has suffered from a major depression or other emotional or mental disorder. The gene—known as 5-HTTLPR—is believed to affect the way a person responds to light. It was discovered by scientists at the National Institute of Mental Health. It comes in short and long versions. The short version lacks some of the components that make up DNA, the material that contains the blueprint for all genes.

A study of 165 people showed that 75 percent of people with SAD had at least one short copy of the gene. People with two short copies of the gene were much more likely to suffer from SAD than those with long versions. Of nonsufferers, about half had two copies of the long gene and half had two short copies or a long and a short copy. Another study of 200 people also showed that those with SAD were more likely to have a short version of the gene.

These findings do not mean that everyone with short copies of the gene will develop SAD. It may take an environmental factor to trigger the condition, such as an exceptionally bad winter or spending large amounts of time in a poorly lit environment.

Another study, conducted at the University of Toronto, found a link between a gene for tryptophan (an amino acid that is converted into serotonin) and SAD. Although the findings are preliminary, the study suggests that tryptophan—which becomes serotonin in the body—might help people with SAD (see Chapter 10 for more on this topic).

Is SAD Adaptive?

Animals either hibernate or are generally less active in winter. Similarly, at least nine out of ten people feel they eat and sleep more in winter. It is normal to undergo some response to seasonal changes, and mild hibernating behavior is one such response that is quite common. So, is SAD in part just a natural response to winter, a leftover state inherited from our ancestors to help us conserve energy?

Hibernation allows an animal to use its body's energy reserves at a slower than usual metabolic rate, so it can be most active during the months of abundant food and good weather. Some ecologists refer to hibernation as "time migration." Of course, differences exist between how bears and humans adapt to winter. Bears undergo a drop in body temperature and appetite, whereas people with SAD tend to eat more. For this reason some have argued that SAD is a failure to adapt, or else an adaptation process that has failed or stopped halfway. We retain some aspects of hibernation behaviors, such as sleeping more, but not others.

Life Events and Stress as Triggers

Some psychologists do not view SAD as a disease, but as a social condition in people with stronger seasonal awareness than others who may suffer from the restrictions imposed by society. According to this view, it is the demands of modern life that result in SAD—i.e., the fact that we still have to get up and go to work or school when our primitive instinct would be just to laze around and eat.

Stress can trigger depression, be it classical depression or SAD. Some people have found that a stressful situation *plus* the onset of winter are enough to induce symptoms of SAD, though it is up to a doctor to determine exactly what type of depression you have. In SAD, as in clinical depression, events that you might normally handle with ease seem just too much.

Many sufferers have found that SAD first developed after a stressful life crisis that occurred in winter. Examples of such life crises might include divorce, loss of a job, bereavement, or a new baby. Someone who has previously shown only very mild symptoms of SAD may develop severe symptoms if put under stress.

Too much stress certainly does not help SAD sufferers; therefore, it may make sense to take steps to reduce stress.

Who Does SAD Affect?

SAD can affect anyone. However, research suggests that certain groups of people may be more vulnerable to developing the condition than others. In particular, women are affected more than men, possibly because of hormonal factors, and women with PMS (premenstrual syndrome) seem to be a particular risk group. Research suggests that SAD may be related to other disorders, especially alcoholism, addiction, posttraumatic stress, and eating disorders, such as anorexia and bulimia. However, SAD has also been reported in children.

As well as having *links* with other conditions, SAD can also be confused with other ailments, such as a viral illness or chronic fatigue syndrome. That is why it is important to get a doctor's opinion to make sure you are not suffering from another problem before you try the suggestions outlined in this book. If your ailment is, for example, glandular fever, light therapy will offer little or no relief. Bear in mind, too, that prolonged fatigue and depression may be symptoms of a wide range of conditions, from diabetes to anemia. SAD may also be confused with allergic reactions, with sleep disorders, or with simple depression.

Let's take a look at how SAD affects certain groups of people, and how it affects and is affected by certain other health problems.

Women

Women are three times more likely to develop SAD than men. The reason for this sex-based difference isn't clear, but according to Dr. Norman Rosenthal it may be linked to female sex hormones. This theory is backed up by the fact that SAD decreases among postmenopausal women.

Sufferers of Premenstrual Syndrome (PMS)

Dr. Rosenthal's work suggests that at least half of all menstruating women with SAD have PMS, with symptoms ranging from irritability and sleep problems to bloating and depression. Some women experience PMS all year, but are more severely affected in winter, while others may have PMS only in the winter.

Many women report similarities between the symptoms of SAD and those of PMS, such as depression, confusion, clumsiness, tiredness, craving for carbohydrates, and weight gain. Research suggests that serotonin levels drop dramatically in some women in the late-luteal (premenstrual) phase, causing these disruptive symptoms. However, the irritability and anger often reported in PMS are more typical of PMS than of SAD. With SAD, people are more likely to suffer from fatigue and lethargy. Furthermore, disturbed sleep is more likely in PMS than in SAD, in which the need for more sleep is the norm.

Sufferers of Postnatal Depression (PND)

There may be a link between SAD and PND. Certainly, women may be more at risk for depression after childbirth, when they may stay inside more and be exposed to less daylight, especially if they have their babies in the autumn. Heather Simons, who has written SAD guidelines for the Cambridge-based organization Outside In (see the Resources at the back of the book), and who has had SAD herself for more than twenty years, believes that many cases of PND are unrecognized SAD. Her advice? "Please, please try to have your babies in the spring!"

Seniors

Older people are at a greater risk of developing SAD because they may be less likely to go out into the daylight. SAD has been linked with a condition prevalent in older people known as *sundowning syndrome* or *sundowner's syndrome*. This syndrome is commonly observed in nursing and retirement homes; it is characterized by an increase in agitation or confusion at the end of the day. Other symptoms include decreased attention, wandering, and possibly hallucinations and illusions. Both having visitors and light therapy improve sundowner's syndrome.

The syndrome has been described as the bane of young doctors who admit a confused older patient in the evening and wait to present him or her to a senior doctor in the morning, only to find that the patient is perfectly well at that time of day! The minor neurological damage from which the person suffers is no problem after a good night's sleep.

Sundowner's syndrome often accompanies Alzheimer's disease. Other causes include illness such as pneumonia or heart attack, side effects of drugs, or any disease affecting the brain directly, such as stroke, seizures, or a tumor. The syndrome has been linked with SAD because it may also occur as a result of disturbances in the circadian rhythms—that is, changes in the sleep/wake cycle, which is controlled by the pineal gland. As mentioned earlier, such changes are thought to be implicated in SAD.

Sundowner's syndrome has been linked with so-called Hesperian depression (named after the Greek goddess of the dusk, Hesperus). Sufferers of this condition show symptoms of SAD in the evening, once the sun goes down. For example, they may be unable to work or to go out once it is dark.

Children

Research suggests that many people with SAD have suffered since childhood. According to the *Journal of the American Academy of Child and Adolescent Psychiatry,* more than one million children in the U.S. may be afflicted.

In a survey of children in a Minnesota school, 6 percent said they experienced extreme mood variations during the winter, with 1 percent reporting outright depression at that time of year. In another study of nearly 2,270 middle-school and high-school students in Washington, more than 3 percent showed symptoms of

SAD. The rate of SAD was found to be higher in teenage girls. The study concluded that between 1.7 percent and 5.5 percent of children between the ages of nine and nineteen may have SAD. It also speculated that there is a relationship between SAD and puberty.

SAD seems to affect not just school performance but general development, including verbal creativity. A large study conducted in schools in Alberta, Canada, found that pupils' performance improved greatly when they were in a classroom that got better light. Over two years, pupils in a classroom with full-spectrum light showed better results in achievement, in rates of attendance, and in growth and development than those in less well lit classrooms. They even had better teeth, with fewer cavities!

How SAD Presents Itself in Children

Two to six percent of children have SAD, the same percentage as are diagnosed with attention-deficit disorder (ADD). Even though the typical age for the onset of SAD is the late twenties, many children experience winter depression, often mistakenly labeled as laziness or a learning disability. Many sufferers, with hindsight, recall their first episodes of SAD as happening in childhood or adolescence. Children (and parents and teachers) may have difficulty recognizing SAD, especially given the lack of public recognition of the relatively new disorder.

SAD in children may take a slightly different form from SAD in adults. Children may be more likely to suffer from fatigue and irritability, or perhaps anxiety, rather than depression as such, though they may be more weepy than usual. They may also experience sleep problems, including disturbed sleep, or the tendency to fall asleep during the day. Their increase in appetite may show as a craving for junk foods or sweets. Some children suffer headaches, perhaps because of the poor sleep and diet. Children may show behavioral difficulties, such as withdrawal from family and friends, crying spells, temper tantrums, and watching more television than usual without really retaining what they have been viewing.

It is easy for both children and parents to miss the symptoms of SAD. So many of the behaviors described above are regarded as "normal" difficulties or teenage moodiness. What child doesn't crave junk food or suffer sleep problems at times? Though children themselves may be aware that something is wrong, they tend to blame the problem on external factors, such as a child or teacher who they perceive is picking on them or treating them unfairly.

When spring comes and the behavior passes, it may be easy to label it as having been "just a phase," to forget all about it and fail to make the connection when trouble arises again at the start of autumn. For that reason it is worth monitoring the symptoms to see if they are seasonal. Does your child behave differently during a winter vacation in the sun or snow? Bear in mind that snow can reflect bright light, and so can lift one's mood even though the sky may not seem sunny. Does your child's academic performance show any seasonal variations, with grades typically dropping in the autumn and winter? Does your child suddenly want to skip out on choir or soccer practice halfway through the autumn term? Does she bow out of going to the disco with her friends on a cold, dark Saturday night?

Other signs of SAD in kids can include poor memory and organizational skills, and difficulty writing, finishing homework, or completing projects. Again, these can indicate a range of other problems, such as attention-deficit disorder, and are fairly typical of many normal children, so it is important to resist jumping to conclusions. However, if SAD rather than something else is the cause, you will find that in spring your child may become more talkative and active, sometimes to the point of hyperactivity, and perhaps be unable to go to sleep early or find that he or she does not sleep well.

The cluster of symptoms exhibited by children with SAD—irritability, bad behavior, and sleepiness—often leads to children being disbelieved or wrongly labeled as lazy or difficult. Undiagnosed SAD—and it often goes completely undiagnosed—can make a child's life a misery and disrupt education, hobbies and

interests, and relationships. Obviously, to make an accurate diagnosis it is crucial to exclude other stresses, such as bullying or a
feeling of being academically pressured at school, as well as illness
or other conditions. Both attention-deficit disorder and clinical
depression may sometimes resemble SAD, but neither condition
should get worse in autumn or winter unless your child has SAD as
well. If you suspect that your child may be suffering from SAD, a
visit to the doctor and a talk with his or her teachers should be
arranged to determine the cause of the problem with certainty.

People Deprived of Light

As explained in Chapter 1, SAD is more common in countries in
northern latitudes because those parts of the world receive less
light in winter. However, people may also develop SAD-type
symptoms in other seasons if they undergo a change in environment that involves their being exposed to less light than before.
Moving to an area that is farther away from the equator, and so
gets less sunlight, may trigger SAD in some individuals. Some people may be affected by a change in their environment or routine—
moving into a home with less light, or changing a work environment (for example, moving from a desk by a window to an indoor
room without windows), or changing work hours so that they go to
work by night. Climate can also have an effect, even when it isn't
actually dark. Fog, for example, can lead to SAD-like symptoms.

Others

Other groups of people have been shown to be more likely to suffer
from SAD than the rest of the population, though comparatively
few studies exist on this issue. More research is needed to clarify
exactly why some people seem to be more vulnerable. These
groups include those mentioned below.

People with Eating Disorders

Individuals with bulimia and anorexia nervosa seem to be more
susceptible to SAD than others. As mentioned earlier, one theory

for why this is so speculates that serotonin plays an important role in both SAD and bulimia nervosa, possibly for genetic reasons. Both disorders are characterized by an increased food intake and a depressed mood. One research project looked at the three components of women's serotonin systems involved in satiety, production of serotonin, and response to drugs that affect serotonin levels, such as Prozac. It was found that women with SAD or bulimia nervosa were more likely to have a particular variation in a serotonin gene called *tryptophan hydroxylase* (TPH).

Research into the possible genetic link between SAD and certain eating disorders is in its early stages, but future studies could have a significant impact on treatment of both disorders, perhaps leading to such developments as new medications targeting serotonin.

Abusers of Alcohol and Drugs

Those who abuse alcohol and drugs are two to three times more likely to develop SAD than those who don't. Experts believe that this correlation, too, may be linked with an inherent lack of serotonin in the brain.

Several studies have linked alcohol cravings to a lack of light. In one such study, a set of rats mysteriously preferred plain water during the week but went for alcohol on weekends. Researchers discovered that, owing to a fault in the timer switch controlling the laboratory lights, the rats were left in complete darkness all weekend. The same finding was replicated and developed in other studies.

People Prone to Depression

People who suffer from depression may be more prone to developing SAD than people who have never suffered from depression. Again, the correlation may be linked to serotonin levels.

Those Whose Culture Demands They Stay Covered Up

People whose culture disallows them from exposing their skin and/or face to the daylight are vulnerable to SAD. Besides the wearing of veils or masks, cultural expectations may include staying indoors a lot of the time, which also cuts down on opportunities to be in the light.

People Giving Up Smoking

Nicotine, like carbohydrates, increases serotonin, while nicotine withdrawal has the opposite effect. As we have seen, low serotonin levels have been linked with SAD.

People with Eye Problems

Partially sighted or blind people may suffer from SAD. However, such individuals can still benefit somewhat from natural light because it reaches the retina. On the other hand, those who have sustained an injury to the eyes, who have certain eye conditions, or who have lost an eye may suffer from SAD. Such individuals may experience SAD throughout more of the year than just winter, because little or no light is being received by the retina at any time of year. Cataracts, for example, cause a narrowing of the lens, thus lessening the amount of light that reaches the retina. For this reason people with cataracts may be at increased risk of SAD.

People Who Wear Dark Glasses

Likewise, dark glasses and sunglasses can trigger SAD because they may block the light from reaching the retina. The benefits of protecting the eyes from UV rays have been well publicized, but for sufferers of SAD a case can be made for taking the glasses off. However, care should still be exercised; one should wear sunglasses when the sun's rays are strong, and only remove them earlier or later in the day.

Is It SAD?

It is possible to have SAD *and* another disorder, such as clinical depression, at the same time, or to have another disorder that may be *confused* with SAD. To reiterate, it is worth checking with your doctor and getting a definite diagnosis before proceeding as if you have SAD.

Fatigue may be a symptom of almost any illness. Most usually, though, SAD can be confused with the following conditions:

◆ Clinical depression;

◆ Hypothyroidism (underactive thyroid), the symptoms of which are feeling sluggish and an intolerance of cold. The thyroid gland produces hormones that regulate the metabolism; abnormalities in the gland can be easily treated with medication;

◆ Hypoglycemia (low blood sugar), which involves feeling weak, shaky, and lightheaded, often with a craving for sweet foods;

◆ Viral conditions. The symptoms of SAD can resemble those of glandular fever (mononucleosis, caused by the Epstein-Barr virus), myalgic encephalomyelitis (ME), chronic fatigue syndrome, or postviral syndrome. Viral conditions tend to be more prevalent in the winter, so it can be confusing and difficult to diagnose the cause conclusively. A consistent history of depression experienced winter after winter may differentiate SAD from these other possibilities. Most viral conditions improve over time with rest and good diet and show up only occasionally, so if the symptoms repeat from year to year, SAD should be considered as a cause;

◆ Sleep disorders, such as sleep apnea (the temporary cessation of breathing during sleep);

◆ Allergic reactions. Pets as well as people spend more time inside the home during winter than in other seasons, so an undetected allergy to cats or dogs may flare up. The symptoms of an allergy will result in poor sleep that, in turn, may be mistaken as SAD;

◆ Iron deficiency anemia.

How Is SAD Diagnosed?

No single clinical test exists for SAD. It is diagnosed on the basis of the patient's medical history, the main clue being whether or not the symptoms are seasonal.

Because an accurate medical history is so important in diagnosing SAD, you can help your doctor by keeping a diary of the symptoms. Points to note include:

◆ **when the depression seems to begin**—some people start to feel apprehensive in August; others may be fine until late November or even December;

◆ **changes in appetite**—whether you eat more or differently;

◆ **changes in sleep**—in particular, whether you crave more sleep than usual;

◆ **whether you have experienced any of these factors in previous years.**

Chapter 5

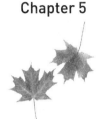

How to Help Yourself:
An Action Plan

The prospect of the gloomy winter months creeping up on you again and again may make you feel powerless, but be encouraged by the knowledge that there are actions you can take to help prevent SAD or to lessen its impact. Before you consider light therapy or antidepressant drugs, both of which are outlined in later chapters, you may find that a few simple lifestyle modifications will help keep SAD at bay, especially in milder cases. This chapter looks at ways in which you can try to preempt SAD and suggests actions to take during the worst days of winter.

If you typically feel more energetic and creative in spring and summer, it may be worth consciously structuring your year around the seasons. Try doing major projects during the seasons that afford more light, and reserving the more routine tasks for the winter. Doing so can give you a greater sense of control and can lessen any guilt involved in letting people down as autumn and winter approach and you feel you cannot honor commitments that are too much for you. In the same way, it may also be a good idea to postpone major life changes until the spring whenever possible. Moving or starting a new job, for example, might be easier to manage in sunnier, warmer weather. Many people do this instinctively, whether or not they have SAD. View autumn and winter as a chance to slow down and allow yourself to take life easier. Slip into a different rhythm from that of the busier days of spring and summer. Go to bed earlier, and accept that you may be less busy or energetic than you are in the summer. It can also help if you try to establish some positive thinking about the seasons so that you can enjoy autumn and winter. Many people associate autumn with fresh starts and a surge of energy after the heat of summer—perhaps as a remnant from school days, when autumn meant the start of a new year. The ancient holiday Samhain, which occurs at the end of October, is a celebration of the start of the Celtic new year, and the Hindu festival of light known as Diwali takes place in November. Why not write down your ten best autumn and winter memories in a beautiful notebook to share with your friends and children? After all, if you have SAD, it may not be the seasons that are your enemy so much as a lack of light, and this can be tackled.

Make the Most of Late Summer

Use the last few weeks of summer to get as much sunlight as possible. For most people, doing so isn't a problem, but others begin to have feelings of impending doom and gloom in August as the light changes, becoming more mellow, with the shadows growing longer. Use these weeks to be outside as much as possible.

You can also use this time to plan for the autumn ahead. Start evaluating your levels and sources of stress, and consider any ways in which they can be minimized. For example, if you have a difficult situation or colleague at work or foresee particular problems, consult with your boss while your energy and coping levels are still high. If you stay at home with children, look at ways to make the daily routine easier. Try leaving a box for shoes in the hall so shoes can't get lost, and pack kids' lunches the night before.

You might also want to consider booking an appointment with your doctor for a general checkup or to talk about or make plans for overcoming winter depression. Your family doctor can be a source of support. Even if no medication is prescribed, it can be helpful to know that you have discussed the possibility with him or her. Points to discuss can include general goals for dealing with the winter months, whether to start light treatment using a dawn simulator or lightbox, and whether drug treatment would be appropriate for you. Your doctor may also be able to refer you to a psychiatrist; since it can take a while for an appointment with a specialist to be scheduled, late summer is a good time to start the process rolling.

You could also research therapists in your area and speak to two or three over the phone. Enter their names, numbers, and your reactions to them in your address book or journal, and have these details ready in case you feel you may need them in the future. See Chapter 10 for more on the topics of drug therapy and psychotherapy as treatments for SAD.

Plan Autumn Activities

Although we opened the chapter by recommending reduced activity in the fall and winter, some people actually find it helpful to attend regular events and to generally stay busy during those seasons. September sees the start of a whole new schedule of day and evening classes, so late summer is the time to consider taking up a new activity to ensure that you are occupied and thus less likely to fall prey to depression. Although many people with winter depression withdraw and don't feel like socializing, company in a structured environment, such as a class, can be less demanding than hanging out with friends. A classroom environment allows you to work away at your woodwork, creative writing, or whatever you fancy without feeling obliged to talk much.

Another option is a group activity, such as singing. The weeks before Christmas, often a difficult period for SAD sufferers, are a busy time for most choirs. Furthermore, singing offers proven health benefits of many kinds. One large Swedish study of more than 12,675 people found that singing in a choir seemed to promote longevity as well as boosting health and mood.

The value of planning is that it helps you feel more in control. Plan something for each weekend of the month. Occupational psychologist Cary Cooper says, "Having something to look forward to, like a matinee movie or concert, is one of the best ways of raising well-being and efficiency."
Make the most of the holiday entertainment season. Feeling isolated can be a dangerous aspect of depression. It is hard to bear in mind that changes in brain chemicals rather than social reality may be responsible for this feeling. Arranging regular companionship can combat this feeling. Get together with another friend who hates winter, and encourage each other to go out, stick to an exercise plan, or contact other SAD sufferers. (See "Resources," at the back of the book, for contact information for a support organization for SAD; in addition, the women's website www.ivillage.com sponsors a SAD message board.)

Think Ahead about Your Winter Routine

Many people find mundane chores such as cooking and cleaning more of an effort in the winter, so plan ways to save yourself energy. Here are some ideas for doing so:

◆ Do your major food shopping on the Internet. Some people find that doing this once every two weeks or with a friend makes delivery charges more manageable.

◆ Consider investing in having someone help you with cleaning or ironing; even once or twice a month needn't cost too much and may make a difference in your level of coping.

◆ Cook several meals in advance on weekends when you have more time, or in early autumn when you feel more energetic. For example, a half gallon of marinara sauce can be frozen in separate portions to serve with a pasta meal or to top a pizza. Or make a big pot of hearty soup or chili and freeze it in individual servings for cold winter nights.

◆ Buy any items you need for your winter wardrobe when they first appear in the stores in early autumn, before you get too lethargic to bother with shopping. Make sure you have enough warm socks, tights, sweaters, and other items. Many SAD sufferers feel better when they take care to stay extra warm (see the section titled "Keep Warm," on page 66).

◆ Invest in extra help with child care.

Be Prepared for the Holidays

Christmas can be a stressful event at the best of times, but if you have SAD, you may find it overwhelming. You have several options. One is not to bother with Christmas at all. *Mary* and her family, who were Quakers, didn't celebrate Christmas with gifts, cards, and festive meals.

> We made a decision early in our marriage simply not to "do" Christmas. The children have never known any different, and I don't think they quite know what people are going on about when the Christmas fuss starts.
>
> I find managing daily life hard enough in the depths of winter, and Christmas seems so complicated! People send us cards, which is quite nice, though I always feel a bit guilty, but then I think, "Oh well, I can make it up to those people all the rest of the year." And in a week or so everyone has forgotten about it anyway, so it makes no difference. Christmas is a peculiar time bubble.

Even if you don't want to do away with celebrating Christmas entirely, you may want to consider scaling it way back. Holiday depression can be made worse by putting pressure on ourselves to live up to unrealistic standards. Is it really necessary to send Christmas cards to dozens of folks? Or to buy a gift for every friend and coworker? Or to decorate the entire house in a manner worthy of Martha Stewart? Or to bake six different kinds of cookies? Consider decorating a small tree and skipping the outdoor lights, or simplifying your gift-giving routine.

Another option is to prepare for the event while your energy levels are still high—in late summer if it suits you. Some people buy presents all year round, whenever they see them. It may be worth clearing a drawer or shelf especially for Christmas and putting bargains away there. Another idea is to shop online or by catalog starting in late summer. *Jane* finds this approach helpful. The holidays are a time of year when she saves herself from as much stress as possible.

> I've learned to buy Christmas cards the minute they appear in the stores. This seems to happen earlier each year, which in a way is quite good for someone with SAD! I even buy the stamps and put them on the envelopes, then I put everything away to be sent in December. I used to write a short newsletter and print out a copy to put into each card. Over the past couple of years, though, I've dropped this and now just copy a short e-mail to everyone.
>
> On Christmas day itself, we eat very simply. I don't invite hordes of draining relatives, and we often go out to a hotel for dinner. I'd love to go to Paris for Christmas but haven't felt up to it yet.

Monitor Your Moods

Instead of simply waiting for your spirits to sink at the end of summer, try to take preemptive action. Remaining aware of your moods means you can stay a step ahead of them instead of being totally at their mercy. One idea is to keep a diary or mood chart, listing your moods and any factors that seem to trigger them. For example, a gray morning may leave you feeling down, especially if you have overslept, realize you have forgotten to run an important errand, have received only bills in the mail, and must rush off to work.

Ensuring that you have a quiet five minutes every morning for meditation or to sort out your thoughts can help. So can writing positive affirmations, such as, "I can manage, whatever the circumstances." Positive affirmations are a powerful tool. The principle behind them is that imagining something to be true will help to create it in your physical reality. For that reason, be sure to say or write affirmations in the present tense (e.g., "I am filled with serenity and peace, no matter what's going on around me") rather than in the future tense ("Everything will turn out just fine"). If they're set in the future, then that will be your reality—you'll tend to view peace and contentment (or whatever you're imagining) as something that will come to you at a later date rather than creating it right now. Likewise, frame affirmations in the positive ("I now experience wonderful health") rather than in the negative ("I am no longer sick").

Keep an eye open for the symptoms of depression. A frequent comment from people with depression is that they find themselves in the middle of it without seeing it coming. You might want to make your own checklist, since warning signs can differ from person to person, or ask your partner or a friend to let you know when they notice changes. Often others are better than we are at seeing that something is not quite right.

Signs that can indicate depression include:

◆ undue pessimism

◆ lack of motivation

◆ low self-esteem

◆ withdrawal from others and feeling isolated

◆ feeling guilty

◆ feeling irritable

◆ feeling overwhelmed and unable to cope

As *Alison* says:

I certainly don't always realize that I'm "going down." I am aware of being grouchy and of blaming everyone around me for everything, but I'm not really aware of how negative I am until others challenge it—and it can take a bold person! One morning I criticized the entire bureaucratic system, from education to the trains to the postal service, and after a short pause my partner said, "Do you have anything good to say about anything?" That made us both laugh, and I realized how irrational my thinking had become.

Monitor Your Energy Levels

In the same way, keep an eye on how energetic you are feeling. When your energy seems to start trailing off, you can steer a path between trying to raise energy levels and adapting to a quieter lifestyle.

Ways to raise energy levels include:

◆ diet (see Chapter 8)

◆ exercise (see Chapter 9)

◆ light therapy (see Chapter 7)

◆ exposure to more daylight (see this chapter and Chapter 2)

As suggested above, keep a diary or day planner—this time for planning the months to come. Consider invitations before accepting them. If someone calls wanting you to do something, ask if you can call them back in a few hours, and use that time to think through whether you can comfortably manage what is involved. An autumn weekend with friends, running a booth at the school Christmas fair, helping to plan a friend's surprise party—all these things may take up energy that, at this time of year, you feel you want to keep for other activities. There is no harm in saying no, either in advance or later on, if you feel you have overcommitted yourself. You can always undertake new projects or honor social obligations in spring or summer.

Organize Your Memory

Poor memory can be a particular problem for some people with SAD. Try to find one simple way to organize your day planner. A large chart or calendar on the wall or using an electronic personal organizer may help.

Katy kept an electronic organizer on her at all times and immediately entered anything into it as it crossed her mind, even if she was walking down the street. She found that if she wrote things down she was 98 percent certain to accomplish them. If you go the electronic route, however, don't forget to keep a supply of replacement batteries on hand!

Mary keeps a small diary with birthdays, appointments, and so on written in it; this method offers the bonus of not relying on batteries. *Jayne* uses a box of index cards on which she's written names and addresses. She found it hard to remember to use a diary or electronic organizer, whereas the index box sits on her desk so she can use it as she works.

Get More Natural Light

Even in winter or on dark days, you can enjoy the health-giving qualities of daylight by getting outside for as little as twenty minutes a day. Here are some ideas to help you plan to do so, as well as some pointers for getting the most out of those wonderful sunny days:

◆ Aim to spend at least an hour outside each day, whatever the weather. Break the time up into smaller portions if doing so is more convenient than going out for the whole hour at once.

◆ In cities such as Seattle, where it rains and is chilly or downright cold for several months of the year, many people manage even in foul weather to commute by bicycle to work and to enjoy the out-of-doors in other ways. If you don't live in the Sun Belt, you can still get outside even in inclement weather, and you'll almost certainly feel better for having done so. Purchase the right gear: a waterproof or insulated parka, gloves, head covering, thermal socks, waterproof shoes, and even waterproof pants, if you wish. If you can't afford expensive new winter wear, you can easily find these items at the local thrift stores. Now bundle up and get outside!

- Go for a walk in the park or around your neighborhood for twenty to thirty minutes to raise your serotonin levels. Surprisingly, even a cloudy winter's day in the U.K. provides 10,000 lux of natural light. The light striking the retina activates the pineal gland, which in turn controls production of the energizing hormone serotonin.

- When you are at work, get outside at lunchtime. Generally make the most of any opportunity to be outside.

- If you wear glasses, remove them, if you can, for at least twenty minutes (longer if possible). Eyeglasses, and especially sunglasses, can block the entry of sunlight into the eyes and slow down its effects on the body.

- If you cannot get out, and if the weather permits, spend some time sitting by an open window. The window needs to be open because glass absorbs UV light, denying you those beneficial rays that activate vitamin D.

- Some research has suggested that certain suntan lotions may be linked with cancer. According to the U.S. Food and Drug Administration, fourteen out of seventeen lotions contain suspected carcinogens in the form of PABA (para-aminobenzoic acid). However, some authorities believe that allergies to PABA are more of an issue than the risk of cancer. To be on the safe side, use a PABA-free or chemical-free lotion. Depending on what type of skin you have, try also allowing yourself some time in the sun without suntan lotion. You can wear a long-sleeved top, wide-brimmed hat, and long pants to protect your skin.

- Never look directly at the sun.

◆ Avoid exposure when the sun is at its strongest—usually between 11:00 A.M. and 2:00 P.M.

Lighten Up Your Home and Work Space

Decorate your home to make the most of light and bright colors that reflect the light. Replace regular light bulbs with daylight bulbs that create full-spectrum light (see "Resources" for retailers of such products). Open the curtains and blinds to let natural light into the house, and prune any trees or hedges that block the natural daylight. Also consider putting extra skylights and windows in your home.

At work, try to sit near a window, or at least ensure that the lighting is adequate. If necessary, bring in your own light, preferably fitted with a daylight bulb.

Keep Warm

Many people with SAD (and without!) report feeling better if they stay warm. With this in mind, in late summer think about whether you need to remodel your house to include efficient winter heating. You will feel far more like dealing with such matters in summer than in winter.

◆ Check the insulation beneath the roof, in the walls, and under the floor. Add or replace insulation as necessary.

◆ Next time it rains, check to make sure that no broken roof shingles are letting moisture in.

◆ Run the furnace to make sure it works. Maintaining your heating equipment properly will increase its efficiency: have chimneys cleaned, remove dust from intake vents, and bleed radiators of any excess air.

◆ Consider installing extra radiators or space heaters in cold corners or in rooms you don't use regularly, such as a guest room or loft, to extend liveable areas and make the house generally warmer.

◆ Order firewood, coal, or heating oil early; prices are sometimes cheaper before the autumn season starts.

◆ Consider having double-paned windows installed in some rooms. Besides increasing the energy efficiency of a home, they reduce noise, too. Alternatively, consider other ways to insulate windows; ask your local hardware store for ideas.

◆ Don't skimp on heating. If you don't want to heat the whole house, invest in extra heating for the room you spend most of your time in.

◆ Some people enjoy an electric blanket, but some research has linked prolonged use of them with cancer, especially leukemia. It is believed that they lessen the production of melatonin, which fights cancer. However, new electric blankets, which use modern methods of wiring, may be less risky. If you are concerned, preheat the bed, then switch the blanket off when you are ready to sleep. A traditional hot water bottle is another option, as is simply piling on more cozy blankets.

Sleep Well, but Less

Craving sleep is a symptom of SAD, but it may help to avoid giving in to the craving all the time. Whereas a good night's sleep is essential to a balanced mood, research shows that sometimes restricting excessive sleep can help boost mood and energy levels. Save sleeping late for one day a week, and try to get up at a reasonable hour each morning. You may find waking up easier if you use an alarm clock that works by faking a dawn (more on the benefits of this in Chapter 7).

It may also help to go to bed at roughly the same time each night; doing so is more likely to set your biological clock and lessen the possibility of disturbances to sleep, a factor linked with SAD.

Some people may benefit from taking an afternoon siesta. Research by the Sleep Council has found that 38 percent of us work best in the morning and 41 percent of us in the evening, showing that we have a natural inclination to snooze at midday.

It will be easier to enjoy a good night's sleep if you don't exercise, work, eat a large meal, or drink alcohol shortly before bedtime. Reading by low light and drinking a glass of warm milk may help soothe you to sleep. Sex and chocolate also work well, according to research by the Sleep Council!

Stay Physically Active

Ideally, of course, physical activity should be a year-long part of your life, not something reserved for specific times. However, assess your level of physical activity in late summer and see what you can do to keep busy as the darker days come along. Even gloomy days seem less overpowering if you are out. Consider walking or bicycling to the store or to work. Alternatively, park your car a few blocks away from your destination, and walk the last bit.

Consider Taking a Winter Vacation

Many people with SAD instinctively plan a holiday in the sun when their spirits are likely to be at their lowest ebb, usually around January or February. *Sally* and her family did this:

> Ideally we would travel from December to February. We'd also love to go away for Christmas, but it's too expensive. Prices seem to drop in January, so we go then. We just take a cheap package to the Canary Islands and soak up the sun for two weeks. It's not quite enough to get us through to the very late springs we've been having, but it helps.

Consider Relocating

Moving to a sunnier part of the country may sound extreme, but if you find life a misery for half the year, relocating is an option that deserves to be considered. You will need to think carefully about whether or not the benefits of extra sun will be outweighed by the changes in major life factors, such as your job, family, friends, and culture. First, spend some time assessing how well SAD can be controlled by other means, such as light therapy and warmth.

If you decide to relocate, pay several visits to your chosen locale during winter to ensure that you really will feel better there; if possible, visit for longer than the usual two weeks. Be sure to check the weather conditions all the way through the winter. Going south does not always mean sunny—witness the hurricane season in Florida (a late-summer and early-fall phenomenon). Also, make sure that the summer won't bring more heat or humidity than you can stand. Such conditions are not only uncomfortable but also in some cases can actually trigger summer SAD, a condition, contrary to most seasonal depression, that causes people to feel depressed during the summer (see Chapter 1).

Seek Help, If Necessary

Make the most of the days when you feel better. We all have daily fluctuations in energy, so remind yourself that if you feel low one day, you may be better able to cope the next.

If, despite your best efforts, you find that you cannot manage and that your mood and well-being are sinking, do seek support.

Chapter 6

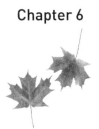

Heliotherapy: A History

In 1905 Einstein put forward his theory of relativity and postulated that light and matter are interchangeable. He wrote, "Light is not just a pleasant side-effect of summer; the whole world runs on light energy."

His words came in the middle of an era when interest in the healing value of light was at its height. Light was used to treat not only depression and other psychological ills, but also a host of physical illnesses. In 1877 it was discovered that sunlight killed the bacteria that caused certain diseases, including tuberculosis (TB), cholera, and anthrax. In those days, TB (also known as consumption) was considered "the captain of the armies of death." Today, anthrax, with the threat of its use in biological warfare, may hold the most immediate terror, but the return of TB in some areas is also a cause for concern.

Over the next thirty years, further scientific research pinpointed UV rays as the "active" part of sunlight's therapeutic effect. In 1903 Danish doctor Niels Finsen was awarded the Nobel Prize for showing that ultraviolet rays were effective against tuberculosis. Sanatoriums such as that of Dr. Auguste Rollier high in the Swiss Alps were established to treat tubercular patients with sunlight. Both children and adult patients were taken outside into the sun for precise periods of exposure, starting with five minutes at a time. Unlike hospitals today, many hospitals built during that

70

era were designed with verandas and French windows to facilitate getting patients outdoors.

Sunlight or UV therapy became widely used for treating many other conditions, including wounds, which healed more quickly and with less scarring when regularly exposed to the sun. Among its many other benefits, sunlight was (and is) also believed to be helpful for preventing osteoporosis and for the immune system. Sunlight was generally seen as good for both physical and psychological health—including depression and lethargy—and the cult of sunbathing began during the early twentieth century.

The discovery of penicillin wiped out not just bacteria but also interest in the medical value of sunlight. Penicillin—so much more dramatic and immediate in its effects than sunlight, and needed urgently in time of war—heralded the start of the drug era. The drug industry grew rapidly, along with the expectation of an instant medical fix and of taking a pill for everything. There were few financial rewards in the relatively time-consuming pursuit of light as a treatment for illness when drugs could do the same thing in less time and for less money. Only recently has the interest in the therapeutic value of light begun to revive. Light therapy for SAD appeared in the 1980s.

Heliotherapy in the Past

Heliotherapy, or sunlight therapy, probably dates back to when primitive man, deeply depressed by yet another chilly night in his cave, emerged each morning to extend his stiff, cold limbs and to feel the sun's healing warmth. In the sixth century B.C., Charaka, an Indian physician, treated a number of diseases with sunlight. Native Americans traditionally use the power of natural elements, including sunlight, in age-old healing rituals. Many other ancient "solar cultures" made use of solariums to stimulate and maximize physical and mental well-being, including the Romans, Incas, Aztecs, Egyptians, and Greeks.

The word *helios* is Greek for *sun*. The ancient Greeks made regular use of sunlight for health purposes. They practiced *arenation* or *heliiosis*: baring the body to sunlight in *aerinaries*, or roofless buildings. Hippocrates and Pythagoras wrote extensively on the use of sunlight in the processes of healing. Herodotus is known as the father of heliotherapy because of his firm belief in the healing properties of the sun. He made regular use of the sun in his own medical practice. "Exposure to the sun is highly necessary for persons whose health is in need of restoring," he wrote. "In every season, the patient should permit the rays of the sun to strike full upon him." Then as now, however, exposure was to be judicious. "But, especially in the summer, this method should be lessened because of the heat," Herodotus adds.

This balanced approach perhaps represents what we should be aiming for today. Sunlight therapy is an area in which excesses can be viewed as a threat. On the one hand, a growing body of scientific opinion purports that the benefits of sunlight to health are being overlooked; on the other hand exists a well-established body of opinion that views UV rays as harmful and the sun as a danger. Such an attitude is reflected in light treatment for SAD: UV rays are routinely screened out of lightboxes.

Another Greek doctor who wrote about sun therapy was Antyllus: "Persons expose themselves to the sun, some cover themselves with oil and others do not; some lie down, resting on sand or a cushion, and some are seated, while others stand or play. This sunlight exposure prevents an increase in body weight and strengthens the muscles. It makes fat disappear. It also reduces hydropic swelling."

These ideas are still under discussion today. A wealth of literature examines the effects of sunlight on the prowess of athletes, and whether muscle growth can be speeded up by sunbathing. (Chapter 2 looks at modern research on the health benefits claimed for sunlight.)

Sun Worship

The world was said to begin with the command, "Let there be light," and there are two hundred references to light in the Bible. In modern Christianity and in much New Age philosophy, light is a metaphor for the sublime, a remnant of the cruder sun worship that prevailed in many cultures from earliest times. Focusing on the power of the sun and often linking reverence for the sun with magic, rather than with religion, occurred very frequently as well.

The ancient Egyptians worshipped the sun god Ra. He was represented by a golden disc, which was also a symbol for the king. The god Apollo represented the sun for the Greeks. The Mayans, located in what is now Mexico and Central America, were renowned for sun worship. They built huge pyramids in its honor. The Incas, who lived in what is now Peru from around A.D. 1200 until the sixteenth century, worshipped the sun god Inti and his wife Kilya, the moon.

In Europe, the early Christian church found it easier to make use of existing traditions—rather than sweep them away and start again—to ensure that its beliefs would be accepted. As James Frazer documents in *The Golden Bough,* the Christmas festival of light was superimposed directly on older pagan celebrations of the reemerging sun. In particular, the old Persian deity of Mithra, who was directly identified as the sun by his worshippers, had become the object of cult worship in late Roman times.

The idea of an infant born around the time of the winter solstice goes back much earlier than Christian times. The day of the winter solstice (December 21) was seen as the nativity of the sun, because the hours of daylight begin to lengthen from that date. The Egyptians, among others, used a baby to represent the newborn sun. "The ritual of the nativity, as it appears to have been celebrated in Syria and Egypt, was remarkable," comments Frazer. "The celebrants retired into certain inner shrines, from which, at midnight, they issued with a loud cry, 'The Virgin has brought forth! The light is waxing!' "

In ancient Britain, worship of the sun was part of early civilization. The massive stones of Stonehenge, arranged on Salisbury Plain between 2000 and 1500 B.C., are aligned to indicate the solstices, the beginning of seasons, and the coming of light, and to predict eclipses of the sun and moon.

The Mesoamerican Mayans in Mexico and Central America tracked the movements of the sun, moon, Venus, and other bodies to create a highly accurate solar calendar. They even built some of their temples, such as Chitzen Itza, to help track these movements as part of their sacred rituals.

The decline of the sun was also marked by ancient peoples. The summer solstice was celebrated by festivals all over Europe from Ireland to Russia. The midsummer fire festivals—marked by huge bonfires, animal sacrifice, and dancing—were the most important of the year among the primitive Aryans of Europe, as they marked the time of year when the sun begins its decline. "Such a moment could not but be regarded with anxiety by primitive man," remarks Frazer. Perhaps our collective memory has inherited some of this angst today. Could it be that hereditary anxiety about the declining sun constitutes a biological basis for SAD?

Research into Light

In 1666 Isaac Newton made the startling discovery that white sunlight was composed of the seven colors of the rainbow, visible to the naked eye when a prism is used to filter the light. Thomas Edison changed night and day for good when he invented the incandescent light bulb in 1879. In many ways we have progressed remarkably slowly since then. So overpowering has been the utilitarian use of light—to extend the day and thus productivity—that more diverse and creative forms of lighting, such as lighting devices for therapy, have only been developed in recent years.

The influence of light and dark on biological rhythms was first described in 1729 by the French astronomer Jean-Jacques de Mairan. His work with the small red flowers of the plant *Kalanchoe blossfeldiana* proved that even plants follow circadian rhythms if they are to flourish. The late nineteenth century saw burgeoning scientific interest in the effects of various colors on plants, animals, and people. Many of the studies took place in the U.S., where in 1876 Augustus Pleasanton used blue light to relax glands, the nervous system, and the organs. Soon thereafter Seth Pancoast used red and blue lights to stimulate and relax the nervous system. Dr. Edwin Babbitt developed the chromodisc for filtering light on to the body. He also pioneered the use of charging water placed in glasses of different colors with sunlight, and using the glasses of water as "solar elixirs."

In the 1920s, Royal R. Rife developed the Rife Beam Ray, designed to destroy bacteria or viruses and diseases, including cancer. His work curing cancer eventually achieved a success rate of more than 90 percent at the University of California. Dinshah Ghadiali developed the spectrochrome, a machine that beamed light of different colors on to different parts of the body. Dr. Harry Riley Spitler, of the College of Syntonic Optometry, developed the use of colored light, delivered into the eyes, to improve vision, balance the nervous system, and achieve other benefits.

Recent Pioneers

The growing interest in sunlight and light therapy in our time can be traced back to several pioneers in the U.S. and Europe who kept going during the years when official medical interest was at its lowest.

John Ott, a Chicago banker, became interested in the impact of light on the growth of plants in 1927 after noting that a pumpkin produced all-male or all-female flowers depending on which type of light it received. Ott went on to research the impact of light on animals. He also founded the Environmental Health and Light Institute and designed indoor lighting that mimics natural light. His work is at the core of much of today's research into SAD.

Dr. Jacob Liberman believes that the dangers of UV rays have been greatly exaggerated and that we are depriving ourselves of their health benefits by hiding behind windows, sunglasses, and chemical sunscreens. (As mentioned earlier, concerns have been raised about PABA-based sunscreens being carcinogenic.) His book *Light: Medicine of the Future* (see "Further Reading," at the back of the book) is a pioneering work on the health-giving value of sunlight and the need for proper artificial lighting.

The Discovery of SAD

Research leading to the identification of SAD began in the U.S. in 1970 when research engineer Herb Kern noticed regular changes in himself during the winter months. Happy and productive in spring and summer, every winter he would become depressed, lethargic, and have problems with his work.

Kern developed a theory that his mood and energy levels were related to the changes in levels of light at different times of the year. He approached scientists working on bodily rhythms at the National Institute of Mental Health, who improvised a lightbox. Within a few days of Kern's undergoing lightbox treatment, his symptoms improved noticeably.

Encouraged, the scientists tried more experiments with light therapy. Each experiment resulted in people's symptoms lessening or even ceasing completely. The discovery of SAD had been made—at the same time as its cure.

SAD was first described and named nearly a decade later by Norman Rosenthal, a doctor from South Africa who studied and worked in the United States, and his colleagues at the NIMH. Rosenthal researched the links between abnormalities in the body's biological clock and depression, and the effects of light on the brain and body.

Rosenthal, like Kern, noticed that his mood and behavior changed during the winter months. His energy levels dropped dramatically, he was filled with foreboding and anxiety, and depression ruled. In spring, his energy and mood soared once more.

Now renowned for his work on the seasons, Dr. Rosenthal eventually traced his own depression to the lack of light during North American winters. His discovery came after he worked with other scientists at the NIMH who had discovered that bright light could stop the production of melatonin at night.

Drawing parallels to the natural seasonal changes in animal behavior and biology, such as hibernation, Rosenthal speculated that depression in winter may be due to human beings' inclination to hibernate. "Perhaps we are closer biologically to our animal brethren than we first thought," he writes.

In the decades since these discoveries, there has been an explosion of interest in and research into SAD. Still, far more study is needed to gain a proper understanding of the condition. We do know that SAD has not sprung up out of the blue. Our need for light is deeply rooted in our biology and our history.

Chapter 7

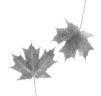

Light Therapy for SAD

Because it isn't always possible to hop on a plane to a sunnier land, phototherapy, or light therapy, is the leading treatment for winter depression. It has a high success rate; around 85 percent of those treated find it helpful. SAD expert Chris Thompson, a professor at the Royal South Hants Hospital, in Southampton, U.K., has found that people are three times more likely to get better if they receive additional light than if they do not. Color-blind (and blind) people respond just as well to the treatment.

A person who undergoes light therapy may avoid the need for drugs, and the treatment has minimal side effects. It does involve some initial expense, and it can be somewhat time-consuming. However, the expense is fairly low, and because modern light treatments are becoming more sophisticated it may be necessary to receive only two sessions per day of twenty to thirty minutes each. For most people the benefits of being free of depression far outweigh these minor disadvantages.

It is possible for a patient to buy and use light-therapy devices on his own; they are much more readily available now than they were even a few years ago. Still, it is recommended that you consult with your doctor before using one, though you may find that some general practitioners know little about light therapy. Light treatment is considered to be relatively safe, but you may benefit more with proper guidance. However, many people can and do use the equipment by themselves. (See "Resources" for a list of retailers of light-therapy devices. To locate a holistic-health practitioner in your area, contact the American Holistic Medicine Association, also listed in "Resources.")

A more important factor to consider in deciding whether to consult with your doctor is the severity of your depression. If you experience serious depression, including feelings that "life isn't worth living," or you cannot complete tasks that are usually routine, then you should consult with your physician as soon as possible. Those with eye problems should also get medical advice before using light treatment.

Indoor Sunshine

The use of "indoor sunshine" has a long history. By the 1890s, European sanatoriums were prescribing incandescent electric "light baths" to treat many physical and psychological conditions. The subject of growing research interest over the past two decades, light therapy is now widely used, in spite of some skepticism from the medical establishment. Indeed, since only an estimated 10 percent of people with SAD have been hospitalized, the condition remains something most doctors haven't witnessed or treated firsthand.

Today, in the coffee bars of Finland, land of the midnight sun as well as of seemingly endless winter nights, you can order a coffee and a "shot" of light—a special bright light at the table to lift your mood. London's Young Vic Theatre introduced its own light café, with large bright-light panels at the tables. Switzerland funds research into light therapy. In Sweden, every building must have a nuclear fallout shelter; all new buildings, including churches, contain cellars incorporating thick concrete walls and heavy lead-lined doors. However, as the Cold War has receded, and with it the nuclear threat, owners of the buildings housing these cellars have had full-spectrum lights installed in them. You will commonly find Swedish citizens basking in their cellars under their full-spectrum lights.

Germany restricts the use of cool white limited-spectrum fluorescent bulbs in public buildings because of their distorted spectral output. Russia uses light therapy to boost productivity and reduce absenteeism in the workplace. Coal miners must spend half an hour a day unclothed in natural light or under full-spectrum artificial lighting, a regimen that has been shown to prevent and treat black-lung disease. Russian researchers have also documented that the body's tolerance to environmental pollutants and the effectiveness of immunization are increased by exposure to full-spectrum light.

Research by Dr. George Brainard, at the University of Pennsylvania, has shown that people without SAD can dramatically improve their handling of stress under extended work conditions of thirty-hour shifts when exposed to bright, white, fluorescent light. In both Russia and Germany, at work sites where individuals are engaged in shift work, the law mandates that full-spectrum lighting be used. Some American companies have noticed that workers are more productive, more accurate, and less likely to be absent in environments that use this type of lighting.

The benefits of light are not limited to humans. In a zoo in New York state, fertility soared after sunlight-simulating lights were installed in an effort to stop vandalism. Cougars, geese, sheep, deer, bear, wallaby, and the chimpanzee all became pregnant.

Bright-Light Therapy

Bright-light therapy (BLT) is the most established treatment for SAD. It consists of looking at special broad-spectrum bright lights for a period ranging from thirty minutes to three hours a day, generally in the early morning. The treatment is believed to work by reducing or stopping the production of melatonin and stimulating the brain to make more serotonin. The light needs to be especially bright—much brighter than ordinary room lights, which typically emit only 200 to 700 lux. The intensity of light necessary for the treatment of SAD is from 2,500 or 3,500 lux to 10,000 lux.

Light devices are becoming more powerful and portable and less expensive, resulting in increasingly wider use. They usually take the form of a lightbox, though dawn simulators are also becoming popular and seem to be effective (see page 85).

When *Sally* suffered from SAD symptoms, her doctor referred her to a psychiatrist, who recommended daily exposure to bright light.

> It really worked. As the lightbox manufacturers said would happen, within two to three days I started noticing changes. I felt lighter and more energetic, and my food cravings diminished. I had so much more energy. On the third morning I looked out of the window and suddenly thought, "It's quite a nice day; why haven't I taken a walk for so long?" I found myself doing jobs I'd been putting off. I had a lot more interest in making the house nice. I revamped the sitting room, got new curtains and big cushions for the sofa, and generally made the place cozy for the winter. Whereas before I had wanted to stay in bed and just run down to the kitchen for endless snacks, now life expanded.

When *Jon* began using a lightbox, the first change he noticed was that colors seemed brighter.

> I use lightboxes regularly in the autumn and winter. Without lightboxes or some other kind of treatment, my life would just not happen during the winter. I'm taking a very intensive class in the evenings as well as maintaining my day job, and I simply cannot afford to let the time go by while I curl up in a corner, just wanting to sleep and eat, which was what happened before. At the moment I can't afford to let one day go; every moment is vital if I'm to get the qualification I'm aiming for.
>
> When I started using the lightbox, the actual depression took about ten days to lift, but I felt changes in myself well before that. In fact, physically, I felt different every day, and I wasn't quite sure what was going on. Now at the end of a winter's day I am tired, but it's a healthy tiredness that comes from doing things all day—not the unnatural tiredness I experienced before that made everything an effort.

For Jon, light treatment alone was enough. Sally, on the other hand, took action in addition to light therapy to combat her SAD. At work, she rearranged her office so that her chair was closer to the window. She took daily walks to get the benefit of whatever sunlight there was. Although she still looked forward to the spring, she felt relieved that winter had lost its terrible hold on her.

Light-Therapy Devices

Light-therapy devices are readily available for purchase by the consumer, and some health-insurance plans cover them. See "Resources," located at the back of the book, for a list of retailers who sell them. Two kinds of light-therapy devices are the lightbox and the light visor, both discussed below.

The Lightbox

The most common devices used for bright-light therapy are fluorescent lightboxes that produce a light intensity of 2,500 to 10,000 lux at a distance of up to three feet away. A 10,000-lux unit retails for around $250 to $500. Full-spectrum light is unnecessary, as the intensity is the most important factor, but a balanced-spectrum light, minus UV-B emissions, is considered ideal.

Most lightboxes can easily be set up any place where you normally spend some part of your day, such as on a desk, on a dining-room table, or in an exercise room. Small lightboxes are available for taking to work or for use when traveling. Jon gave his father-in-law, who is a writer, a lightbox for Christmas. The father-in-law routinely kept it turned on while he was working, and though he didn't have SAD he said he enjoyed the effect.

As with all light treatment, it is important to avoid looking directly into the lights, as this creates the possibility of eye damage. Some people may be instructed to look at the lightbox briefly at regular intervals, though for many doing so seems to be unnecessary. This is because the light penetrates the eyes obliquely and even passes through closed eyelids.

Some manufacturers of lightboxes will allow a risk-free trial period of two weeks or so, which should be enough time to see if you benefit from the treatment.

Light Visors

Light visors are worn on the head, much like a baseball cap, and deliver the light from above the eyes. They offer the advantages of being more convenient, allowing for mobility and permitting the user to carry on with her normal activities. They produce white light with no UV rays.

The disadvantage of these devices is that they are battery powered, requiring the batteries to be replaced from time to time. Furthermore, they seem to be less powerful and successful than lightboxes. However, some people find that using a visor for just twenty to forty minutes each morning is enough. Others use a combination of visors and boxes to suit their routine.

When to Use the Device

Light therapy is most helpful if used daily in winter, starting in early autumn or even in August for some SAD sufferers. Some work has shown that starting treatment early in the year may help eliminate symptoms altogether, giving the user a SAD-free winter. Conversely, the later light therapy is started, the more time may be needed to see results. Light therapy often starts working within one to three days. If you do not feel any better after two weeks, consult your doctor or other health-care provider for further help.

Most people stop using light therapy in the spring as brighter natural light returns. However, you may continue to benefit from using the lightbox in spring and summer in the event of a sequence of rainy or cloudy days.

Studies show that light therapy is most effective when used in the morning. Most people find that taking a session between 6:00 and 8:00 A.M. works, perhaps with the addition of another session in the afternoon between 3:00 and 7:00 P.M. Be aware, however, that adding an afternoon session can cause insomnia. Some find the use of light therapy before bed helpful, but, again, doing so is likely to cause insomnia in most people.

The more powerful the lightbox, the shorter the session that is needed. Generally, twenty to thirty minutes spent with a lightbox producing 10,000 lux (or one hour a day at 5,000 lux) is the average "dose" that produces positive improvements.

As a rule of thumb, whether you are a morning or an evening person may affect when it is best for you to use light treatment. Here are some guidelines:

◆ **For night owls (or those with DSPS—delayed sleep phase syndrome—to use its medical name):** If you have trouble waking up in the morning and often feel sluggish for hours after awakening, even if you have slept longer than usual, you may benefit from an early morning session, between 6:00 and 8:00 A.M.

◆ **For morning people ("early birds" or those with ASPS—advanced sleep phase syndrome):** If you are at your most alert in the morning, possibly becoming tired around lunchtime, and often go to bed early by choice, you may benefit from a thirty-minute session at 10,000 lux taken between 3:00 and 7:00 P.M. Short, periodic sessions throughout the afternoon at high intensity, or longer exposure at lower intensity may also be considered. You may not benefit from a second session in the morning.

It may take some experimenting to find exactly what time of day suits you best, but generally it is recommended that you take your light medicine at the same time every day.

Once you start feeling better, you may be able to cut down on treatment time or even miss it entirely on some days. Most people seem to be able to miss a couple of days without ill effects, but by the third day without light therapy symptoms may return.

Dawn/Dusk Simulators

A dawn simulator is like an alarm clock that works by faking a dawn. The device emits gradually brightening light for half an hour before the user wakes up. The increasing light suppresses the production of melatonin in a natural way. One advantage of this system is that visual stimulation is a more soothing way to wake up than the traditional shrill alarm clock. Also, unlike audio stimulation, the illusion of dawn helps set our biological clock to awaken at the same time every day.

Research was conducted at the New York State Psychiatric Institute to find the effect on SAD of dawn and dusk conditions. A computer was used to simulate the gradual appearance of dawn and the gradual disappearance of light in the evening in a pattern characteristic of spring. (During the winter months, by contrast, the light disappears and appears fairly abruptly.) When subjected to this gradual, simulated dawn, SAD sufferers reported improvement as substantial as if they were receiving full phototherapy. Blood tests revealed that dawn simulation resulted in cutting off the production of melatonin and restoring the circadian rhythm. When exposed to the artificial dusk simulation, the patients experienced good, deep sleep. They described it as almost like "a pleasant hypnotic sensation."

The simulation of dawn and dusk has great potential in the treatment of SAD, and more work is proceeding along these lines. The simulators are based on the premise that our ancestors awoke according to the rhythms of natural light (although farm workers past and present have always gotten up in the dark to do some chores by lamplight).

Dawn/dusk simulators appear to be most effective for those with mild symptoms, those who did not succeed with bright-light therapy, and those who have had success with bright-light therapy but still experience difficulty waking up. However, some people have found the simulators to be as effective as light treatment, if not more so, and feel the benefits immediately. The simulators may be particularly good for teenagers who dislike hanging around in front of a lightbox and who have difficulty waking up. One study showed that twelve out of twelve teenagers found it easier to wake up with a dawn simulator (and their parents agreed). The devices may also help to improve the quality of sleep. Another study showed that people who used them fell asleep sooner the following night.

Rachel, a twenty-seven-year-old lawyer, had suffered depression, which she called a "predictable darkness," all winter long every year since age seventeen. She also got hungrier than usual and tended to crave sweets in the evening. In spite of sleeping for ten or eleven hours, she still felt tired during the day and lost interest in her usual activities. She often felt irritable, worthless, and guilty, she didn't want to see her friends, and her sex drive was very low.

After three weeks of using a dawn simulator, Rachel felt much better. Her mood was "almost as good as in the summer," and she had far more energy. Her appetite returned to normal, she slept less, and she was much more productive at work.

Paul, a fifty-three-year-old who complained of depression from November to April, recalled having endured winter depression for almost twenty years. In addition to feeling down, Paul lost pleasure in most everyday activities. He craved food much more, ate more, and usually put on about twenty pounds each winter. Paul often woke during the night and was unable to fall back to sleep for several hours. He would get out of bed and spend hours reading or surfing the Net. He was often tired during the day and had trouble concentrating on tasks such as work and reading the newspaper. He tended to be more tense and irritable during the winter and more likely to worry about his physical health.

Paul undertook dawn-simulation therapy at home. After three weeks, his mood improved, he regained interest in his work and other activities, and he was able to sleep through the night. His appetite was still a little greater than in the summer, but overall he felt much better.

Which Therapy?

Researcher David Avery found that lightbox therapy led to an 80 percent reduction in symptoms, a dawn simulator 70 percent, Prozac 55 percent, and evening light therapy 33 percent. Generally, lightboxes are regarded as more powerful and effective than visors, though visors are more convenient. Dawn simulators are the most convenient form of light therapy since they work while you sleep.

Jon used the visor in the morning when he first woke up; he wore it for twenty minutes while lying in bed chatting with his wife. He also used a 10,000-lux lightbox, which he considered more powerful, at 4:30 in the afternoon for thirty minutes. Because he was taking a class, there was always reading to catch up on; using the lightbox gave him a convenient time to do so. Or sometimes he would "stare into the box and use the time to chill out and just relax." Jon notes that people without seasonal depression dislike the light and find it irritating. His wife complained that it gave her a headache, whereas he "soaked it up."

Marta came to the U.K. from Brazil and found herself falling into the familiar pattern of SAD sufferers: in September and October she would begin to feel very down. She thought it was because she had come from a naturally sunny country to a darker, colder one, and she supposed that SAD was something that only affected people from sunny countries. That was until she made friends with *Alison* (mentioned in Chapter 1), who also suffered from SAD. Marta used a lightbox to treat her condition, and Alison used a visor. The two swapped treatments for a while and found little difference in their effectiveness.

When Light Therapy Doesn't Work

Some people may find that they are not helped by bright-light therapy. There are various reasons for this. It could be because they are not using the equipment properly. If your use of a light-therapy device seems to be ineffective, contact your doctor and/or the manufacturers of the device to discuss how you are using it. Talking to someone from a support organization may also help; often a layperson who uses the device on a daily basis can offer insights that might be unknown to or overlooked by a professional. (See "Resources," at the back of the book, for organizations that might be able to put you in touch with other SAD sufferers.)

Alternatively, perhaps your depression has nothing to do with SAD, even though the condition may appear to be seasonal or to actually become worse in winter. Some people spend more time in the house during winter, consequently experiencing social isolation and depression. Or perhaps you're suffering from chronic depression for which other treatment is needed. Clinical depression may fail to respond to bright-light therapy—or at least to bright-light therapy alone. A study at the University of Alberta, Canada, showed that people recovering from severe depression recovered in 16.9 days if they were in a sunny ward, but took 19.5 days if they were in a dimly lit ward—a difference of 2.6 days. However, these patients also received other treatment for depression, including antidepressants and counseling. If light therapy fails to benefit you, it is important to consult your doctor. Sometimes light therapy works better when combined with other treatments.

Julie found that a lightbox helped, but only when she used it in combination with antidepressant medication during winter (she took Cipramil). This regimen helped her make it through the winters, but she did not feel it was a proper substitute for sunlight and only felt like herself when spring came again and she could halt her medication.

Carole suffered depression as well as SAD and took antidepressants year-round, adding treatment with a light visor during the darker months. She also attended a support group for people with depression and received some counseling.

Safety and Side Effects

As stated repeatedly throughout this book, it is worth consulting with your doctor before using light therapy to rule out the possibility that you have clinical depression. Clinical depression can easily be treated with modern medications and/or counseling, but it won't respond to light therapy.

In addition, you should check with your doctor before starting light therapy if you have any of the following conditions:

◆ an eye disorder, such as glaucoma, cataracts, or detached retina

◆ any sort of depression that lasts the entire year, even if it gets worse in winter

◆ a rash, high temperature, or any other symptoms of illness, in which case you might have an infection

◆ another condition that necessitates taking medication. Some drugs can make you photosensitive, as can contact lenses, in which case you may need to start on a lower "dose" of light treatment

Research seems to indicate that UV rays are not essential in light treatment; indeed, they are generally screened out of light-therapy equipment, or reduced to low, safe levels. Generally, light therapy is considered a safe form of treatment, with mild, temporary side effects experienced only by a minority. Irritability, agitation or excitability, slight nausea, mild headache, and eyestrain for the first few days appear to be the main side effects. These can be reduced by sitting farther away from the light, or by reducing the length of the session time, or both. Consistent, long-term overuse may arouse mania or feelings of being "high" in a tiny proportion (around 1 percent) of users.

If you are on antidepressants, it may be possible to reduce the dose of the drug once light therapy has been established and proven effective. Again, consult your doctor about the best way to do this; reducing or giving up medication without medical supervision can be dangerous.

Can Light Treatment Help Other Conditions?

Another recent use of light therapy, developed for the military, involves shining light onto a nonvisual part of the retina to prevent sleepiness over a period of forty-eight hours. In addition, the shining of a strobe light in a sleeper's eyes has been found to stop snoring. However, these and other nontherapeutic uses of light are hardly to be applauded as they will lead to imbalances in the body and thus potentially to health problems.

Many impressive medical uses of light exist, but we shall focus here on its applications in complementary or alternative medicine. These include the following:

- Ultraviolet light is used to treat psoriasis.

- Full-spectrum or blue light cures jaundice in newborns by chemically breaking down excess bilirubin in the skin.

- Another study showed that abstinent alcoholics who received light therapy in the form of a dawn simulator found it easier to stay sober, raising the possibility that light therapy might be used to help treat those who abuse drugs and alcohol.

- Some research suggests that keeping a light on all night in the middle of the menstrual cycle may help to normalize long menstrual cycles (those lasting more than thirty-four days).

Although the claims for light therapy are far ranging, the area needs more research since many of the studies on its effectiveness have been small and haven't been replicated.

Other Types of Light Therapy

At the moment, light therapy for SAD is administered via the eyes to activate the pineal gland. However, one study showed that it is possible to alter a person's circadian rhythm by shining light on the back of the knees, suggesting that treatment via the skin might be a possibility for the future.

Colored-light therapy, introduced in the United States in the nineteenth century, still remains experimental and has undergone far less research than bright-light therapy. However, the use of specific frequencies of light is proving to be effective in treating a growing number of conditions. Whether SAD is one of them remains to be seen.

Other types of light therapy include brief strobic photostimulation (BSP), which is exposure to rhythmically pulsing colored light. It is often used together with other forms of therapy, such as counseling, to treat painful emotional states such as anger and tension.

Colored strobe-light therapy is used as an adjunct to psychotherapy and to enhance vision and learning ability. This type of light therapy should only be conducted by a qualified therapist or doctor. Such therapies are not usually recommended for people with SAD. Bright-light treatment, which counters the light deprivation associated with winter, remains the most effective and best-researched treatment to date.

Colored-light therapy often blends into color therapy. Color therapy is based on the theory that certain colors are believed to possess certain properties that affect the individual in specific ways. Red is believed to stimulate the nervous system, an effect that raises a person's readiness for action. Blue is supposed to help lower blood pressure and induce calm. Certain colors are used routinely in public life, such as Baker-Miller pink, a shade of pink used in prisons and other institutions to reduce aggression and violence. Much more research is needed to assess the impact of color on people with SAD.

There are other light therapies that blend into complementary therapies. Laserpuncture is an offshoot of acupuncture, a branch of traditional Chinese medicine that uses needles to stimulate acupuncture points all over the body. Developed in Russia, laser-puncture uses low-energy laser beams instead of needles to stimulate the acupuncture points. Laserpuncture may help with conditions that worsen SAD, such as stress, but the therapy has not been definitively tested as a treatment for SAD itself.

Chapter 8

Nutrition and SAD

Can eating the right foods help to rebalance a person's brain chemicals and boost his or her mood? Yes, according to some specialists in nutrition. Their suggestions fall in line with the latest thinking on healthy eating and form a diet plan that can be followed year-round for optimum health.

As discussed, people with SAD tend to crave and overindulge in simple carbohydrates—both sweets and starches—and may put on weight in winter. Any annual weight gain needs to be monitored since staying within reasonable weight limits is important for a person's overall long-term health. Emotional or comfort eating—that is, eating in response to difficult situations, anxiety, depression, or loneliness—is also common in SAD sufferers. So for people with SAD, it is important to plan what to eat and when.

Since bingeing on simple carbohydrates can increase certain brain chemicals such as serotonin, the urge to do so is thought to be a form of self-medication. The problem with simple carbohydrates, including white bread, white pasta, pastries, and other sweets, is that their effect is temporary and leads to further cravings for the same kinds of foods. Many nutritionists believe that by balancing protein and complex carbohydrates a person can raise levels of serotonin via his diet and build a more resilient brain chemistry that will help him resist cravings and the urge to overeat. This chapter looks at some suggestions for monitoring diet so as to control mood and cravings.

Winter Weight Gain and How to Tackle It

It is worth looking at the issue of winter weight gain squarely in the face. Though the phenomenon is dispiriting, it is possible to do something about it.

In evolutionary terms, storing fat in the body for winter made sense; for our ancestors it could have made the difference between survival and death. Many centuries ago, when food was scarce in cold weather, the shortening days were a signal to the body to slow down its metabolism and start storing fat for the winter. Less light and lowered levels of serotonin also set up a craving for carbohydrates, which increased insulin levels. Higher levels of insulin helped to store energy (calories) in the fat cells (i.e., to increase stores of fat), and also lowered blood sugar, thus increasing hunger. This combination was an effective survival technique in the cold. The extra carbohydrates were mopped up by our bodies' striving to keep warm in the millennia before central heating, and by the physical labor we had to perform for everyday survival tasks.

Nowadays, however, instead of food being scarce in winter, the Western world sees the arrival during that season of the biggest eating event of the year: Christmas (and Thanksgiving in the U.S. and Canada). Instead of living off our stored body fat as we chop wood, hunt, and beat our laundry clean in the stream, we all too easily spend time adding to those fat stores while driving to work or sitting in front of the TV. In addition to the ready availability of food, the cold and dark mitigate against our going out for exercise. The result: weight gain.

The problem with winter weight gain is that it is not always lost during the summer—or at least not completely. Over the years, this has a cumulative effect. For example, if you gain ten pounds each winter and lose eight pounds each summer, you are still gaining two pounds each year. That's an extra twelve pounds every six years, which adds up to a health threat that deserves to be considered carefully.

The good news is that winter weight gain can be tackled as part of a year-long eating plan that aims to address cravings. The key to doing so, according to the latest research, is a combination of protein and complex carbohydrates.

The Protein-and-Carbohydrate Combination: Why Your Brain Needs It

By understanding more about how food affects the brain, and by practicing a few basic healthy principles of nutrition, it is possible to gain more control over your eating. Essentially, different types of foods work on different brain chemicals.

Protein

Protein feeds your body the amino acid tryptophan (among other amino acids), which is then used by the brain to make serotonin. Foods rich in tryptophan include any protein, such as chicken, turkey, red meat, milk and other dairy products, fish, eggs, beans, and legumes. If you are watching your weight, choose poultry, lean meat, fish, and low-fat cheeses, such as cottage cheese, feta, and Edam. Goat's cheese, cheddar, and parmesan all have a high fat content.

Protein has a number of other functions that help stabilize body chemistry. For one, it boosts production of dopamine, another of the brain chemicals thought to be lacking in people with SAD. Dopamine helps us initiate movement and express emotions. Protein also helps stabilize blood-sugar levels.

Carbohydrates

Boosting serotonin levels is more than a matter of simply going on a high-protein diet. Your body also needs carbohydrates, because they help tryptophan to pass into the brain via the bloodstream. A key point here is that the carbohydrate you choose should be the complex or unrefined variety, such as that contained in potatoes, whole-wheat or multigrain bread, oats, brown rice, and whole-wheat pasta. If you are being careful about your weight, eating lots of vegetables will give you the carbohydrates you need without adding too many calories. Try to avoid simple carbohydrates, such as those contained in cakes, cookies, candy, and other sweets. Simple sugars do not have a long-term effect on serotonin because they can boost insulin too much, causing a rebound of low blood sugar and, in turn, lowered levels of insulin. Also limit your intake of refined white flour, white rice, and other refined grains. They bear a similar effect on the body as that of simple sugars: boosting insulin levels quickly, which causes the system to "crash" when blood-sugar levels fall.

A combination of carbohydrates and proteins is needed to help balance mood, though if you have SAD you may need more carbohydrates than most people in order to boost serotonin levels enough.

The Sugar and Alcohol Factors

Research suggests that people with SAD appear to process sugar differently in winter than they do in summer or after light therapy in winter. Given the craving for sweets experienced by so many people with SAD and the links between alcoholism and SAD (see Chapter 4)—and the fact that a lack of serotonin is implicated in both conditions—it is interesting to consider the work of Kathleen DesMaisons here. A specialist in sugar and alcohol addiction, Dr. DesMaisons has worked out an eating plan designed to combat cravings for sugar and alcohol and to naturally boost levels of the brain chemicals serotonin, dopamine, and beta-endorphin.

It is Dr. DesMaisons' belief that people who crave sugar or alcohol probably have an inherent extra need for serotonin. They may also lack other brain chemicals, including dopamine and beta-endorphin. Both sugar and alcohol cause a release of the neurotransmitter beta-endorphin, which produces a sense of well-being. According to Dr. DesMaisons, people with certain brain chemistries respond to the effects of sugar more significantly than other people. She explains the mechanisms that lead to imbalances of brain chemicals, such as "priming," whereby eating or drinking a small amount of a substance (like sugar) can make a person want more of the substance. In summary, the more sugar is eaten, the more beta-endorphin is released, causing the brain to compensate for this "excess" by shutting down some of its beta-endorphin receptors. The result is low beta-endorphin levels, which may cause feelings of depression, tearfulness, and low self-esteem, as well as a further craving for sweets.

To combat low levels of serotonin and other brain chemicals, Dr. DesMaisons suggests the following regimen:

- Keep a food diary.
- Have a breakfast that includes protein.
- Eat three meals a day.
- Eat protein with every meal.
- Eat complex carbohydrates.
- Reduce or eliminate sugar and simple carbohydrates.
- Consider cutting down or eliminating alcohol (besides being full of sugar, it is a natural depressant).
- Eat a small baked potato (with its skin) as a prebedtime snack to boost insulin production, which in turn helps raise serotonin levels while you sleep. Eat it without protein—say, with margarine or olive oil rather than cheese—since protein interferes with the serotonin-building process.

The rest of this chapter examines some of these suggestions, as well as suggestions from other nutritionists. For a more detailed discussion of the use of nutrition to combat depression, read Dr. DesMaisons' book *Potatoes Not Prozac*, listed in "Further Reading," at the back of the book.

Eat Breakfast

It is well documented that people who eat food totaling two thousand calories in the morning lose an average of two pounds per week, while those who eat the same number of calories after 6:00 P.M. gain weight. Breakfast kick-starts your metabolism, which tends to slow down in winter. On top of the wintertime reduction in metabolism, when you skip breakfast you give your brain the message that you are in starvation mode. As a result your metabolism slows down even more to conserve the body's fat stores as much as possible.

Try eating a combination of protein and complex carbohydrates at breakfast, along with some fresh fruit or juice for vitamins, minerals, and antioxidants. If you've breakfasted on nothing but toast and coffee for years, it may be a bit of an effort to make the change, but your physiology will probably appreciate the results. Chances are you will feel fuller, more energetic, and less likely to crave sugary snacks at midmorning. Here are some suggestions for breakfast:

- hash browns and a poached egg, scrambled egg, or omelet
- oatmeal or other hot cereal with skim or low-fat milk and a handful of raspberries or blackberries (these fruits are recommended because they're low in sugar, but choose another favorite fruit if you prefer)
- a mixture of raw oats, sunflower seeds, half a chopped banana, and skim milk or plain yogurt
- turkey bacon and whole-wheat toast plus sliced tomato
- hummus on a bagel
- low-fat cottage cheese with chopped fruit
- two slices of whole-wheat or multigrain toast with peanut butter
- two hard-boiled eggs, a slice of whole-wheat toast, and a citrus-fruit salad, such as grapefruit and/or orange

- whole-wheat pita bread stuffed with Edam cheese and lettuce or tomato
- whole-wheat pancake with chopped fresh fruit and yogurt

The Importance of Food Planning

For people with SAD, planning what and when to eat can be especially helpful. This includes thinking ahead to times when you know you will be vulnerable. For example, if a workday lunch means indulging in fatty or sugary foods, you may be better off taking raw vegetables and cottage cheese to nibble.

Plan your shopping so that you head straight for the healthy foods, and ignore the aisles that stock cookies and cakes. The old advice to avoid shopping when you're hungry may not apply here. If you go to the grocery store and you're hungry, focus on how good and fresh those vegetables and other healthy foods will taste once you get them back home. Bear in mind the habit factor, too—it is supposed to take thirty days to change a habit!

Coping with Cravings

Once you are eating three meals a day with a good balance of protein and complex carbohydrates, you may find that cravings diminish of their own accord. Here are a few more tips to help you win your battle against the urge to overeat.

- Increase your protein intake. Although you may be eating protein at every meal, you still may not be getting enough for your needs. Sometimes extra protein can help fend off cravings for less healthy foods.

- Eat a small amount of what you want when you want it. Eating one to three pieces of chocolate when you crave it may satisfy your sweet tooth, whereas fighting the craving can lead to overeating later on. Nutritionist and author Debra Waterhouse (see "Further Reading," at the back of the book) says that eating small amounts of the food we crave can help balance brain chemicals and boost serotonin levels. On the other hand, other nutritionists disagree, saying that a little now may lead to a lot later. Another idea is to keep sugar and simple carbohydrates as part of regular meals, eating them as dessert or with a protein. It's a matter of finding out what suits you. If a little chocolate leads to a binge, it may be better to avoid it altogether.

◆ Rest. You may be confusing hunger with tiredness.

◆ Distract yourself. Try to keep busy if you feel a craving coming on. Call a friend, read a book, or do some task around the house.

◆ Try to wait for twenty minutes before giving in. Then wait another ten minutes.

◆ A technique from Ayurvedic medicine suggests drinking a mug of hot water with a little lemon or lime juice and a teaspoon of honey stirred into it to see if what you're experiencing is emotional "hunger" or real hunger. If you are not really hungry, lemon tea can give you a taste of sweetness and may help fill you up.

◆ Schedule your cravings. For example, if you know you tend to binge in the evening, set out one portion of the food you're going to allow yourself—a slice of chocolate cake, say—and allow yourself to enjoy it. Back it up with healthy nibbles, such as grapes or carrot sticks.

◆ Identify your danger times. Common low points are midafternoon around 4:00 P.M. and evenings. Then, change your routine accordingly. Arrange to meet a friend or go out.

◆ Try to identify any emotional sources of eating and deal with them. Look at situations and stresses that make it more likely you'll eat or that may trigger you into comfort eating, such as when you're busy at work or alone.

To Snack or Not to Snack

Given that many people with SAD experience the urge to nibble, what about snacks? Do they have a role in a healthy diet? There is a case for and a case against snacking.

If one nibble leads to another and then another, and snacking fails to satisfy the uncontrollable hunger that some people with SAD report, it may be better to try and stick to just three meals a day, plus a snack of complex carbohydrates at bedtime. Schooling your body to wait for meals may, after a few days, help lessen the feeling of round-the-clock hunger.

On the other hand, some nutritionists believe that snacks are important. They maintain that people should eat every three to four hours to keep brain chemicals and blood sugar boosted, and thereby avoid tiredness, irritability, and overeating later. If you tend to suffer from premenstrual tension, consuming carbohydrate snacks no more than three hours apart may be especially important to help maintain your blood-sugar levels.

Find out what suits you. The type of food you snack on is just as important as what you eat at mealtimes. Try to avoid sugar, which may indeed lead to more eating than you had planned. Bear in mind that snacks do not have to be huge; sometimes a couple of crackers may be enough. Try eating just half of what you feel you want to eat.

Healthy snacks include:

- the breakfast suggestions given above
- half of an egg-salad sandwich on whole-grain bread with lettuce and tomato
- rye crackers with low-fat cheese
- a tortilla wrap with chopped tomato, salsa, and Edam cheese
- fruit
- seeds

- a handful of almonds and two dried figs or apricots

- apple slices and cheese sticks

- a baked potato with tuna fish and cottage cheese, or hummus and a grating of Edam, or tomato with chopped onion and a touch of chili

- a whole-grain bagel with low-fat cream cheese and salmon

- whole-grain pita bread with canned black beans, olives, feta cheese, and lettuce

- instant soups or meals (those to which you just add boiling water), such as pea or lentil soup

Slightly Reduce Caloric Intake

Starving yourself is not only painful but also ineffective. As with missing breakfast, starving yourself sends a message to your body that it is vital to hang on to fat stores. Your metabolism then slows down, and you keep the fat instead of losing it.

However, cutting down your caloric intake just a little will work over time. It is surprisingly easy to shave calories off your daily intake so that you hardly realize it is happening. For example, skipping a single cracker or cookie can save around seventy calories, while avoiding a glass of wine saves a hundred calories. Eating your toast without margarine or butter saves around seventy calories a slice. Even if you make such reductions only once a day, what you don't eat can amount to quite a bit of weight lost in the course of a year.

Other Dietary Changes to Help You Feel Better

- Cut down on or avoid coffee and other caffeinated beverages, such as tea and soft drinks. Several studies have linked depression with a high intake of caffeine. They show that depressed patients tend to consume fairly large amounts of caffeine; and the higher the intake, the more severe the depression. If you drink four or more cups of coffee or servings of soda per day, try substituting decaffeinated coffee, herbal tea, or mineral water.

◆ Avoid processed foods that contain artificial coloring and preservatives.

◆ Pay attention to your body to determine if any foods cause allergic reactions, tiredness, heaviness, digestive upsets, or any other adverse reactions. Keeping a food diary will help with this project.

◆ Eat oily fish, such as tuna, salmon, or herring, once or twice a week. Oily fish is rich in the omega-3 type of polyunsaturated fat. Low levels of this fat may increase one's vulnerability to depression.

◆ Eat a balanced, varied diet that includes plenty of fresh fruits and vegetables (at least five servings daily from the fruit and vegetable group) to ensure that you get most of the vitamins and minerals you need. In addition, taking a multivitamin and mineral supplement will provide a good nutritional basis and prevent any imbalances from depleting your body of any one vital substance. However, remember that vitamin and mineral supplements are not meant to replace a healthy diet. They work in conjunction with foods, not in place of foods. You won't benefit from skipping breakfast or lunch and swallowing a handful of pills. Individual supplement needs are best discussed with a qualified health practitioner, such as a nutritionist, but supplementation specifically for SAD is discussed in Chapter 10.

Chapter 9

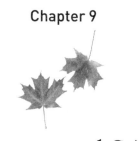

Exercise and SAD

After light therapy, exercise is the most frequently recommended treatment for SAD, especially if it is done in daylight. Exercise treats both body and mind and is well known for its success in alleviating many forms of depression. One study found that exercising for two hours a day in the early morning led to significant improvement in people with SAD. Luckily, this level of exercise may be unnecessary in order to benefit. You don't have to spend hours in the gym or start running marathons to experience improvement in your SAD symptoms. Recent thinking on exercise maintains that brisk walking and simply getting more physical activity into your daily life can be beneficial. This is good news, given that the last thing most SAD sufferers feel like doing is vigorous physical activity. *Jon* and *Marta* bear this out:

> Normally, I love exercise; I work out regularly at the gym, do weight training, and swim three times a week with my wife. But when I was in the grip of SAD, I just couldn't do it. I was too tired—exhausted all the time. Until I underwent light therapy, I just couldn't get started on any exercise. — *Jon*

> Walking kept me going while I was in the depths of depression. No matter how bad I felt, I always felt a tiny bit better if I got outside and went for a walk in the fresh air. Once the antidepressants kicked in, my energy came back and I wanted to be

with people, so I joined an evening yoga group. That would
have been unthinkable with SAD. — Marta

Marta's and Jon's words highlight the fact that, for people with
SAD, exercise may be more effective if it is combined with some
other kind of treatment. Many SAD patients combine exercise
with other forms of help, such as medication, light therapy, and
changes to their diet. However, given the power of exercise to
affect mood, any amount you can manage is worth trying. People
who lead inactive lives are twice as likely to suffer depression.

The majority of the physiological benefits of exercise start
kicking in after just a few days. These benefits are immense. As
well as banishing depression, regular exercise has been linked with
a lower risk of breast cancer, reduction in the risk of stroke, and a
boost to the immune system. Exercise stimulates the thyroid
gland, improving its functioning and thus making the metabolism
work more effectively. Regular exercise reduces appetite and so
makes a person less likely to binge on carbohydrates.

Long-term regular exercise, along with the right diet, is enormously helpful in preventing obesity. It also reduces the incidence
of type-2 diabetes by at least a third. Individuals who become and
remain overweight as a result of SAD are at increased risk of diabetes and other health conditions. Exercise can also help lower
blood pressure, help with efforts to quit smoking, raise HDL
(good) cholesterol, promote bone health, and reduce the risk of
some cancers. Last but not least for SAD sufferers, regular exercise
helps people sleep better.

Alison found that once she got started on light therapy and
took up swimming again, her sleeping improved enormously.

> I would fall asleep very naturally and sleep deeply and well, but
> without that feeling of heaviness I used to have. Waking up was
> a pleasure. I'd lie in bed and listen to the wind or the rain or
> whatever and would feel quite nice and cozy, like it was good to
> be alive. I wouldn't have that awful feeling of, "Oh no, another
> day, how am I going to get up?"

Exercise in the Daylight

A number of studies have shown that, for people with SAD, exercising in the daylight is the key factor in improving mood. In a preliminary study of women with SAD, exercising while exposed to daylight was more likely to be associated with fewer seasonal depressive symptoms than was exercising with little light exposure.

In another controlled study, 120 people who worked indoors were tested to see what was most effective at improving depression and other aspects of health. They performed fitness training two or three times a week while exposed to either bright light (2,500–4,000 lux) or ordinary light (400–600 lux). Compared to relaxation training, which was used as a placebo (something that was not meant to have any effect), exercise in bright light improved general mental health, social functioning, symptoms of depression, and vitality, while exercise in ordinary light improved only vitality.

Even when it's cloudy outside you will still benefit from exercising in the daylight. Remember from previous chapters that exposure to daylight—not just sunlight—can help boost levels of serotonin and so make you feel better. Opportunities for exercising out-of-doors are obviously reduced in winter, but there are ways to manage it. Short bursts of activity work best for some people—a brisk ten-minute walk in the morning, at lunchtime, and again in the afternoon, or a longer twenty- to thirty-minute walk at lunchtime. Outfit yourself with appropriate cold-weather clothes that keep you warm and dry even in winter weather. If you can't manage to get outside, try to exercise near a window, a bright lamp, or your lightbox, if you have one.

Getting Started

It is important to realize that you can start feeling better after even one exercise session. Researchers at Indiana University found a significant lessening of depression that lasted for at least two hours after moderate exercise. This shows that any kind of exercise is better than none. If you feel very lethargic, try to increase your daily activity levels by a small amount—even five minutes a day to start with.

Experts recommend getting at least thirty minutes of moderate to intense physical activity most days of the week, and preferably daily. Research also shows that half an hour of aerobic exercise four times a week will help banish depression. Spread out over a day, thirty minutes is actually relatively little exercise. And your activity needn't be strenuous or involve expensive equipment or special clothing. It can be accomplished simply by taking three brisk ten-minute walks, which you can build into your everyday activities, such as walking up the street to mail a letter. Set small, easily achievable goals on a daily basis.

Suggestions for other easy ways to start exercising include the following:

- **Walk the children to school**—it's good for them, too.

- **Wash the car**—park it up the street so you have to walk to and fro with buckets of water.

- **Walk to the store and back**—carrying a couple of bags increases your activity level, but to avoid straining your back they shouldn't be too heavy.

- **Play actively with your children**—get a ball and spend ten minutes in the yard or park.

- **Garden**—when autumn sets in, prepare for spring by spreading mulch, planting bulbs, or raking fallen leaves. If your local ordinances allow it, build a bonfire as a reward for your labors.

- **Park a few blocks away from work or shopping, and walk the rest of the way.**

- **Clean the house**—this is especially effective if you move from task to task as vigorously as possible. For example, vacuum the floors, then clean the bathroom immediately afterward.

◆ **Use the house as a gym**—run up and down the stairs while tidying up; put items away as you come across them rather than placing them all at the bottom of the stairs to be taken upstairs later.

◆ **Reduce the amount of time you spend watching TV, or at least do something physical during every commercial.**

◆ **Create an exercise mentality**—do this in very small steps by leaving your exercise clothes and shoes on the bed or by the back door and putting them on when you arise in the morning. Even if you end up not doing any exercise, you have still taken one small step toward a more active lifestyle.

◆ **Find excuses to visit people**—walking to see a friend can be a very effective antidepressant. See if you can find a book to lend or a jar of homemade jam to share from those late summer days when you had more energy. Or just drop in without an excuse.

◆ **Push back the barriers of "being tired"**—after doing your ten minutes or so of activity, see if you can push yourself to continue for another five minutes. Increase the increments progressively until both your body and mind become used to exercise.

How Exercise Helps Improve Mood

The effect of exercise, as we have seen, is to improve mood. It can achieve this as effectively as antidepressants in some cases, a fact that is well documented. Exercise stimulates the brain to release hormones called *endorphins*, the body's natural painkillers, which produce a sense of well-being. Endorphin production usually begins about fifteen to twenty minutes into an exercise session and peaks after about forty-five minutes.

Physical activity is also thought to produce other important effects on the brain. As well as improving mood, exercise boosts blood flow and oxygen supply to the brain and so speeds up brain activity. This is important given the role played in SAD by certain brain chemicals and by the circadian rhythm (the twenty-four-hour biological clock).

A U.S. Surgeon General's report contained the finding that, just as changes in brain chemistry can affect behavior, so changes in behavior can affect brain chemistry. Studies with animals suggest that permanent structural changes in the brain—including extra blood vessels and nerve endings—can result from regular exercise. It has also been found that brain-wave activity is positively altered by exercise training and good physical fitness.

Although more research is needed before the influence of exercise on the brain is fully understood, we know that disturbances of brain chemicals such as serotonin and dopamine have been implicated in depression. Exercise may help to normalize brain concentrations of these chemicals, so logic as well as experience point to exercise as good medicine for those with SAD.

What Type of Exercise?

As mentioned earlier, exercising in the light has been pinpointed as important for those with SAD. Research also suggests that aerobic activities improve mental health for people with SAD. Repetitive movements—such as walking, running, and cycling—increase levels of serotonin, so those types of activities are important in the treatment of SAD.

For overall fitness, experts recommend a program that incorporates aerobic activities as well as activities to promote strength and flexibility. Aerobic activities, such as walking briskly or jogging, are those that speed up heart rate and breathing. They increase cardiovascular fitness and endurance. Activities that build strength and flexibility both improve muscular endurance and mobility (important for everyday activities) and help to maintain bone density (important for the prevention of osteoporosis). They include such activities as carrying shopping bags, lifting weights, stretching, dancing, and yoga.

The best kind of exercise, though, is really the kind you enjoy best. If you look forward to your workout, then you are most likely to keep it up. You also need to consider other factors, such as how sociable you are feeling. Would you be more motivated and have more fun exercising with other people? Or would you prefer to go it alone? Finally, an exercise program needs to fit easily into your routine—an important consideration on a dark winter's night when you don't feel like going out.

Once You're Exercising

Once you've gotten going, you may want to progress to an activity that is closer to a formal exercise routine—one that is moderately more demanding in terms of discipline and physical requirements, but that is still compatible with the level of energy you want to expend. Here are some ideas:

◆ **Stretching**—SAD and winter often involve a lot of huddling up to keep warm; stretching gives your body a chance to work out its kinks and remove any tension. If you don't fancy yoga, Pilates is very easy and safe. Consult a local health club, community center, library, or the Yellow Pages for listings of books, videos, and classes.

◆ **Cycling**—Instead of driving, ride your bike for those short runs to the stores or to visit people. Bicycling also offers the advantage of being outside.

◆ **Dancing**—Dance classes come in all shapes and sizes, from ballroom to Latin American, from line dancing to flamenco, from tap to jazz to funk. Some communities offer dance-therapy classes or dance and drama classes that can be used therapeutically or simply as a means of self-expression. Ask your local health club or community center for details. Alternatively, you could always simply put on some music, open the curtains, and dance at home.

◆ **Exercising with friends**—Get a group of friends together in the park and play Frisbee, or organize a trip to the nearest ice-skating rink. Exercising in a group for fun is far more effective than slogging it out alone. Doing so may also make you stick to your plan rather than give yourself excuses for not doing it.

◆ **Swimming**—Since warmth seems to help SAD sufferers, ask around or experiment to find out which is the warmest pool near you, then swim a few laps.

◆ **Rebounding**—Jumping up and down on a small trampoline in the privacy of your own home is easy to fit into most routines and may be less daunting than fancier gear such as an exercise bike. It is also very helpful for kick-starting your metabolism. Inexpensive bouncers are easily available and can be used for five to ten minutes or more while watching the news or a favorite TV program.

◆ **Floating**—If you don't feel like swimming, try floating. Research shows that time spent in a flotation tank benefits both hemispheres of the brain, making you more creative, more imaginative, and better able to solve problems. It is also proven to be good for addictive behaviors, which could be helpful if you have been struggling with overeating. To locate a flotation tank, ask at your local fitness center or medical center, or see the Resources section at the back of the book.

◆ **Videocassettes and DVDs**—For those chilly days when you just can't bring yourself to go outside, try exercising to a videocassette or DVD. A tremendously wide variety of exercise videos is available—everything from yoga to kickboxing to weight training to dance aerobics. Try a few from the selection at your local library or video store to find one you enjoy. Ask a friend to join you.

◆ **Weight training**—If you want to exercise more seriously, weight training burns more calories per minute of exercise than aerobic exercise, and the effect on the metabolism lasts longer. With weight training, the increased activity of your metabolism lasts for minutes or even hours after you stop exercising. Over weeks or months, your general metabolic rate increases.

What about Calories?

Calories can be a bit of a dirty word in fitness circles, as can *weight*. Counting calories and trying to burn off a set number of calories or a certain amount of weight is rather frowned on by many fitness and nutrition experts. Such a strategy is thought of as being old-fashioned, ineffective, and as putting too much pressure on people to set impossible goals and lose unrealistic amounts of weight. It is far better to think in terms of creating a long-term healthier lifestyle that incorporates exercise as a natural part of it.

That said, many people still think in terms of calories, and many fitness and weight-loss centers offer calorie counters to help customers gauge the amount of exercise required to burn a certain number of calories (see chart below). If counting calories is not taken too far, it can be a helpful way to take the weight-loss bull by the horns.

To lose one pound of body weight, an individual needs to burn thirty-five hundred calories more than she takes in. This may sound daunting, but let's revisit the suggestion that you spend half an hour a day engaged in brisk walking, perhaps broken down into three ten-minute sessions. Such a regimen alone is enough to burn one thousand calories in a week.

How Many Calories Are You Burning?

Here are some examples of the average number of calories burned by a person weighing 150 pounds doing various types of moderate to intense activity:

Activity	Calories burned per hour
Bicycling at 6 mph (9.6 kph)	240
Bicycling at 12 mph (19.3 kph)	410
Jogging at 5 mph (8 kph)	740
Jogging at 7 mph (11 kph)	920
Running in place	650
Running at 10 mph (16 kph)	1,280
Swimming at 25 yards/min. (22.8 m/min.)	275
Swimming at 50 yards/min. (45.7 m/min.)	500
Tennis (singles)	400
Walking at 2 mph (3.2 kph)	240
Walking at 3 mph (4.8 kph)	320
Walking at 4 mph (6.4 kph)	440

Obviously, weight loss will be speeded up if you reduce the numbers of calories you take in at mealtimes and in between. It is far harder to lose calories by exercising than it is to consume them. Just think: walking for an hour burns about the same number of calories as are provided by two slices of bread and butter! (Advice for controlling cravings and eating a balanced diet is given in Chapter 8.)

Chapter 10

Other Treatments

Light therapy is the treatment of choice for SAD, but a minority of people find that it doesn't help them. Some individuals find that light therapy works better in combination with other treatments. Preliminary trials have pointed to a number of remedies as being potentially helpful for SAD, and to others as less helpful. More research is needed to determine which are truly effective. This chapter examines several of these potential treatments.

Drug Therapy

How effective are antidepressants? Many of the SAD patients we interviewed for this book said that antidepressants had revolutionized their lives. Some used medications for a short while, just to "get them out of the hole"; others relied on antidepressants longer term. Medication may be more effective when used in combination with light therapy.

Jon tried antidepressants for three years before discovering light therapy. He thereafter gave up his medication because he felt well enough using extra light alone. *Marta* took antidepressants in autumn and winter only. *Carole* took medication year-round since she suffered from clinical depression as well as SAD. *Sally* took antidepressants for five months one autumn, but felt so much better after realizing what was going on and adjusting her lifestyle accordingly that the following year she no longer needed them.

Some controversy exists as to whether antidepressants really work, or whether the improvements are due to the placebo effect (all in the mind). Some research has shown that so-called active placebos (which mimic the side effects of antidepressants, such as causing dry mouth and insomnia, but contain no actual antidepressant) work as effectively as real antidepressants. It has also been found that reading self-help books (like this one!) can be as effective as antidepressants—and works faster.

That said, the modern pharmaceuticals that are generally used for depression treat the serotonergic pathways of the brain and thereby raise levels of the neurochemical serotonin. The most commonly prescribed drugs for SAD are called *selective serotonin-reuptake inhibitors* (SSRIs). They include the drugs fluoxetine (Prozac), paroxetine (Paxil), and sertraline (Zoloft). They may produce fewer side effects than older-style antidepressants, but can still cause some, such as anxiety, upset stomach, headache, insomnia, and others. Tricyclic antidepressants and monoamine oxidase inhibitors have also been used successfully in the treatment of SAD, but generally people experience more side effects with these drugs.

Psychotherapy

Psychotherapy is usually used concurrently with other forms of therapy in the treatment of SAD. The patient and his therapist set goals based on the patient's individual needs.

Forms of talk therapy that can be helpful include behavioral therapy, which may focus on unhelpful behavior patterns (such as not paying bills when feeling depressed), and insight-orientated treatment, a long-term approach that focuses on resolving psychological conflicts. The latter can be extremely helpful to those suffering from SAD or, indeed, from any form of depression. Family and couples therapy may be helpful because of the impact of SAD on people close to those afflicted with it.

Cognitive therapy—often recommended for people with SAD—seeks to help people change how they think about things. It focuses on identifying and challenging rigid, negative beliefs or inner dialogues the patient may be unaware of. By using techniques to challenge a depressed person's assumptions, the therapist helps to change or modify his thinking. An example of an unhelpful or unrealistic view might be "Everyone should like me." The therapy would focus on learning to modify the belief to something along the lines of "I enjoy people liking me, but I realize it's not always going to happen."

Cognitive therapy explores the role of faulty or negative thinking in making people anxious or depressed and suggests a way to recover from such thought patterns, via cognitive restructuring. According to Aaron Beck, who formulated key components of cognitive therapy, the ways in which we process information are governed by structures called *schemata*. These schemata are made up of rules for explaining incoming information and can have a powerful effect on how we experience and relate to the world. Treatment consists of correcting illogical schemata with new information that challenges these deep-seated beliefs.

Biofeedback

Biofeedback, as the name suggests, is a technique that gives a person extra feedback about the state her body is in. It aims to "tap into" connections in the brain between many different areas that are not usually taken advantage of, and thus to help the patient gain more control of automatic functions, such as heart rate, breathing, body-fluid regulation, and regulation of temperature and blood flow.

The feedback can take the form of an audible tone that varies in pitch, lights that turn on and off, or a line on a computer screen. A common form of biofeedback, EMG biofeedback, provides the person with feedback on how tense her muscles are. If computerized biofeedback equipment is used, a line or other image representing the patient's muscle tension is produced on a screen. The therapist then helps the patient relax her muscles; the patient can see the progress for herself by watching the computer image change. She then works on improving her response.

Vitamin D

As explained in Chapter 2, vitamin D is well known for its effects in helping to maintain normal calcium levels. In addition, vitamin D exerts an influence on the brain, spinal cord, and hormone-producing tissues that may be important in the regulation of mood. One study found that mood improved in healthy people without SAD who received 400 or 800 IU per day of vitamin D for five days in late winter. However, vitamin D supplements have not been shown to help people with SAD, according to the small amount of research that has been done on the subject. A large study of women found that supplementation with 400 IU per day of vitamin D had no impact on the incidence of winter depression. Also, no difference in vitamin D levels has been observed between people with SAD and those without it. Furthermore, the antidepressant activity of light therapy has been shown to be independent of changes in levels of vitamin D. So the benefits of extra vitamin D in treating SAD remain unproven.

It is probably best to avoid experimenting with vitamin D supplementation in hopes that it might help your SAD symptoms, as vitamin D is toxic if taken in excess. Whereas 400 to 800 IU daily is a relatively safe dose, vitamin D is not easily eliminated from the body. The body's own synthesis of the vitamin, on the other hand, is self-regulating. It is much easier and safer (and cheaper) to boost bodily levels of vitamin D simply by getting more daylight.

Vitamin D is available in some foods; the richest sources include cod liver oil and oily fish, such as sardines, herring, mackerel, tuna, salmon, and pilchard. Fortified dairy products are another good source. Eggs, liver, and butter provide a little.

Vitamin B-12

Depression can be one of the first symptoms of vitamin B-12 deficiency, so supplementation of this vitamin has been recommended
for SAD. However, one clinical study found that vitamin B-12 (as
cyanocobalamin) worked no better than a placebo in a double-
blind trial. (*Double-blind* means neither the subjects nor the clini-
cians administering the study knew who was taking vitamin B-12
and who was taking the placebo.) Another study, however, suggested that vitamin B-12 might work better if the daily dosage was
divided into three smaller doses rather than taken all at once.

It is always better to take any B vitamins as part of a vitamin-B
complex, to avoid imbalances, or as a natural supplement in the
form of brewer's yeast. Food sources of B vitamins include oats,
green leafy vegetables, legumes, whole grains and cereals, fortified
breakfast cereals, fish, and meat.

L-Tryptophan

Serotonin itself cannot be taken in supplement form because it is
actually produced in the brain. Even if serotonin supplements
were taken, the substance cannot be transported into the brain via
the bloodstream. However, the substance the brain uses to make
serotonin—the amino acid tryptophan—can be taken in supplement form.

A number of medical trials have shown that removing L-tryptophan from the diets of SAD patients who are feeling better in
the summer or after light therapy brings about a relapse into a
depressed state. These results suggest that taking supplements of
tryptophan might be helpful.

In another, small trial, 4 to 6 grams of L-tryptophan given in
divided doses daily was as effective as light therapy in treating
SAD. It has been suggested that L-tryptophan may be of particular use to people who fail to benefit from light therapy. It has
also been shown to help those who are already receiving light
therapy.

The acronym 5-HTP stands for 5-*hydroxytryptophan*, which is a substance related to L-tryptophan that also increases serotonin production. It has been used for its antidepressant effects. Although no research data is currently available on the efficacy of 5-HTP in treating SAD, it may prove to be useful for the condition. If you decide to try 5-HTP, stick to the recommended dosage, as nausea can be a side effect.

Melatonin

Because changes in melatonin levels are believed to be an important factor in SAD, experimentation has taken place to see if supplements of the substance could help in treating SAD.

Some work has suggested that a small dose of melatonin (0.25 mg) taken about eight hours after waking may help to regularize sleeping and waking patterns and the circadian rhythm. On the whole, however, melatonin has been found to be ineffective and may even make things worse for people with SAD, reversing the benefits of light therapy and actually adding to the sluggish feeling sufferers find hard to take.

St. John's Wort

According to research projects involving people suffering from SAD, taking St. John's wort (*Hypericum perforatum*) has resulted in around a 40 percent improvement in symptoms. Some of this may be due to a placebo effect (believing it will make you feel better makes you feel better). It may be more effective if taken in conjunction with light therapy.

An herb well known for its antidepressant effect, St. John's wort has a long history. The ancient Greeks believed that it had supernatural powers and that its fragrance caused evil spirits to fly away. The Romans must have been of the same view; they burned its leaves and flowers on Midsummer Day to rid them of evil spirits.

The plant was later adopted into the Christian world when someone realized that it bloomed close to John the Baptist's birthday (June 24). The black marks on the leaves were said to be a symbol of his beheading at the insistence of Herod's daughter, Salome.

St. John's wort has undergone trials as a treatment for SAD. In one uncontrolled trial, people were given 900 mg per day as well as either bright-light therapy (3,000 lux for two hours) or dim-light therapy (300 lux for two hours—a placebo). Both groups experienced significant improvement in their symptoms of depression. The study's authors concluded that St. John's wort was beneficial with or without bright-light therapy, but a placebo effect of the herb itself cannot be ruled out in this study.

In another uncontrolled study, three hundred SAD patients were asked if they reported overall improvement in their depression while taking St. John's wort. Some used light therapy as well as St. John's wort, and they reported more improvement in sleep quality than individuals using the herb alone, but overall their improvement was not significantly different from that of subjects using only the herb.

More clinical trials are needed to clarify just how helpful St. John's wort can be for SAD, but anecdotal evidence suggests that many people not only find it useful but rely on it to some extent. How much of this is a placebo effect or psychological dependence and how much is a real improvement isn't clear.

If you decide to try St. John's wort, be aware that any improvement in your depression may not be noticeable for a week or two. Also be aware that you should avoid exposure to the sun while taking St. John's wort; the herb can cause photosensitivity in direct sunlight. If you are taking any medication, you must check with your doctor before taking St. John's wort; it interacts with some drugs, primarily including indinavir, warfarin, cyclosporin, digoxin, and theophylline. St. John's wort may also interact with a wide range of other drugs, including oral contraceptives, anticonvulsants, SSRIs, and triptan (used for migraine), so get advice before taking the herb.

Aromatherapy

The aromas of many essential oils are used as antidepressants, including jasmine, rose, neroli, rosemary, melissa (lemon balm), and lavender.

Aromatherapy combined with light therapy may help treat SAD, according to work by psychiatrist Teodor Postolache. He suggests that there are links between the sense of smell and SAD. Dr. Postolache found that the more depressed SAD patients felt, the less accurate they were at identifying smells. However, in summer, they had a more acute sense of smell than people without SAD, suggesting a link between SAD and the sense of smell.

When you breathe in through your nose, the olfactory (smell) nerves are stimulated, triggering a direct pathway to the brain's limbic system, which is involved with memory, emotion, mood, expression, and instinctive behaviors, such as self-preservation. In *psycho-aromatherapy*—the use of aromatherapy to affect the psyche—it's crucial that the odor of the essential oil is welcomed. One study showed that a pleasant odor caused a wave of electrical activity in the right hemisphere of the brain, home of imagination, creativity, and aesthetic awareness. Dr. Postolache found that SAD patients seemed to be particularly unable to identify smells by means of the right nostril (olfactory sensors in the right nostril send messages to the right side of the brain).

A sense of smell plays an important part in many animals' awareness of the seasons. Hamsters largely lose their sense of when to build nests and hibernate if they lack olfactory bulbs. Given the fact that in the long-distant past resting during winter may have been important for survival, Dr. Postolache suggests that as humans evolved we may have lost certain genes, resulting in some loss of awareness of the seasons and of our sense of smell. He speculates that people affected by seasonal changes may have preserved this heightened sense of smell. In other words, SAD sufferers are an evolutionary throwback whose survival mechanisms work too powerfully for the world in which we live today. This theory fits in with the idea of SAD as an exaggerated form of hibernation.

Ionizers

Ionizers are devices that work by releasing negative ions, which are molecules that each contain an extra electron and that help to clean the air. Some research has found that ionizers help to reduce the irritation and depression of SAD while also improving energy levels.

One study on high-density negative ionization for people with SAD showed a 50 percent improvement or more for nearly 60 percent of the subjects who received the high-density ionization. This contrasts markedly with the other group, in which only 15 percent of those receiving low-density ionization experienced 50 percent or greater improvement. There were no side effects, and all of the patients who responded to the therapy relapsed when ionization was discontinued.

Another study showed that high-density ionization was as effective as light therapy in treating SAD. In a third study, however, nearly 61 percent of subjects using light therapy in the mornings completely recovered after four weeks; compare this to the 32 percent who made a complete recovery when they were only exposed to a deactivated negative-ion generator and received no light therapy.

Marie, a forty-five-year-old who for five years had suffered depression from late October until April, was losing interest in most activities, including socializing and sex. As with many SAD sufferers, her appetite grew and she craved heavy foods and sweets in the afternoon. Marie also suffered sleep disturbance. She would wake up in the middle of the night, and feel tired during the day, especially midafternoon, "as if my arms and legs had weights on them."

A friend suggested an ionizer; after two weeks of using it Marie felt much better. Although she couldn't say for sure that her productivity at work was as high as it was in summer, she felt that most of her interest in work, sex, and socializing had returned to normal, along with her appetite, energy levels, and ability to sleep soundly.

Breathing Deeply

Shallow, constricted breathing can be a result of depression or can make it worse by creating an inadequate supply of oxygen in the blood. Deep, regular breathing helps to increase the amount of oxygen that reaches your lungs, blood, organs, and cells. It also relaxes your body and mind.

How to Deepen Your Breathing

- Lie down with your back flat on the floor, your knees bent, and your feet a small distance apart.

- Rest one hand on your stomach and the other hand on your chest.

- Inhale slowly and deeply through your nose, taking the breath into your stomach so that your hand feels your abdomen rise. Your chest should move slightly along with your abdomen. Exhale just as deeply, and feel your abdomen and ribs move.

- Once you are comfortable with this movement, inhale deeply; then blow the air out gently through your mouth.

- Deep-breathe for five to ten minutes once or twice each day. This exercise can be done for up to twenty minutes at a time, whenever you feel the need to relax and focus your energy.

Other Remedies

Many complementary and alternative therapies are available to treat forms of depression. Choosing one is truly a matter of individual taste and experimentation. The following remedies have all been recommended.

- The effect **music** has on physical conditions such as pain, muscle tone, blood pressure, and heart rate is well known.

Music therapy may help people deal with some of the more negative feelings associated with SAD, such as anxiety, morbidity, uncertainty, low self-esteem, and loneliness. Music therapy can take a wide range of forms, including songwriting, singing, playing an instrument, listening, drumming, dance, and musical puppet play.

◆ **Laughter** is said to release endorphins, the brain chemicals that increase feelings of well-being and counteract SAD. The cheap, multipurpose "drug" of laughing has been found to lower blood pressure, reduce stress hormones, increase muscle flexion, and boost immune function. Some hospitals have developed "laughter therapy" programs. In countries such as India, laughing clubs— where members gather in the early morning for the sole purpose of laughing—are becoming popular. While it's difficult to laugh on demand, watching comic videos, enjoying a laugh with a friend, or just trying to see the funny side of life from time to time may all help.

◆ Listen to a tape of **natural sounds,** or look at **pictures of natural vistas** in books or art galleries. According to the Johns Hopkins School of Medicine, natural sounds, such as the gurgle of a brook, and natural sights, such as a mountain panorama, are highly effective at improving mood and can even reduce discomfort during surgery by 43 percent.

◆ Take a **sauna** to remind your body what those hot summer days really feel like. While you're sitting there try to remember last summer in as much detail as possible, and visualize the return of those balmy days; it's only a matter of time before they arrive again. After your sauna, write out your ten best memories of summer in a lovely notebook or on special paper, perhaps to share with your children or a friend.

◆ **Light scented candles, burn oils** with flowery scents, or indulge in bunches of **real flowers** or a fragrant potted plant, such as hyacinth.

◆ **Visualization techniques** can help lift you above your present mood. For example, visualizing a ball of sunshine can help to calm emotions, make you feel happier, and relieve stiff or painful areas, suggests psychologist and hypnotherapist Phyllis Allen of the Derbyshire Royal Infirmary, in England. Try visualization for longer-term purposes, too, such as setting life goals. Close your eyes and relax as much as possible; now ask yourself how you would really like your life to be. Note any images that flash into your mind and write them down. Then, focus on them again in your head in as much detail as possible, to get a clear picture of what you want. At the end of each session, try to make at least one practical move toward achieving your goal. If your dream is to own a house in the country, call a few real-estate agents and have them send you some details, or book a stay in an inn near your area of choice.

◆ In Ayurvedic medicine, depression is seen as losing touch with the freedom of the deep inner self and relating too much to the outside world (an extreme form of "object referral"). Treatment of depression involves working on **rediscovering your inner self**, often through meditation or sitting in quiet thought, perhaps combined with gentle stretching exercises, such as **yoga.**

Conclusion

SAD has more than two decades of clinical research behind it, and public interest in the topic is growing all the time. However, a view of the "winter blues" as a treatable disorder is still regarded by some in the traditional medical community with suspicion, despite clear evidence of the widespread distress caused by the condition. Being affected by the gloom of winter is taken for granted as part of the human condition.

Yet the fundamental physiological facts underpinning SAD cannot be dismissed so easily. The eyes are literally gateways to the mind and the body. The light they absorb triggers vital biological processes, including the ability to wake up and the ability to go to sleep, to name but two. These waking and sleeping rhythms are among the most fundamental of bodily processes; we live our lives by them.

Jacob Liberman describes the eyes as an extension of the brain. He compares their immense complexity (they have more than one billion parts) to that of a space shuttle (with just 5.2 million parts). Unless we are partially or fully blind, around 90 percent of the information we receive comes via the eyes. Of the three billion messages relayed to the brain every second, two billion are sent from the eyes. Our entire blood supply passes through our eyes every two hours; the eyes use a third as much oxygen as the heart. Not just windows to the soul, but also marvelously receptive sensing organs, our eyes are uniquely equipped to take in perhaps our most ignored nutrient: light.

The fact that light fluctuates with the seasons is so basic that we have forgotten about it. We are conscious at some level of light and its waning—hence the depression and other symptoms we experience when we lack light—but we may fail to realize how much we need it. Yet although to some extent we have lost touch with our seasonal nature, we remain seasonal beings.

It is hoped that this book both raises your consciousness about the effects of light and its absence, and inspires you to enjoy the changing seasons and the positive aspects of winter. Take pleasure in an invigorating walk, the crisp beauty of a snowy day, hearty soups and stews, the coziness of a fire. Above all, perhaps, winter offers the opportunity to relax, to slow down. The pressure is off. Take advantage of the opportunity to go to bed early, stay home with the family, or just be alone. The value of this "hibernating" state should not be underestimated, even though it may often be denied. By following some of the suggestions in this book, you will find that a restful winter, in conjunction with a new attitude toward light, will leave you refreshed and ready for the more energetic demands of spring.

Further Reading

Babbitt, Edwin, *Principles of Light and Color* (Citadel, 1967).

Cooper, Primrose, *The Healing Power of Light* (Piatkus, 2000).

DesMaisons, Kathleen, *Potatoes Not Prozac* (Simon and Schuster, 1998).

Downing, Damien, *Day Light Robbery* (Arrow Books, 1998).

Frazer, James, *The Golden Bough* (Macmillan, 1922; Simon and Schuster, 1996).

Hobday, Richard, *The Healing Sun* (Findhorn Press, 2001).

Liberman, Jacob, *Light: Medicine of the Future* (Santa Fe, NM: Bear and Company, 1991; reprinted 1998).

Liberman, Jacob, *Light Years Ahead*, 1992 Conference Report (LYA Publications, 1996).

Liberman, Jacob, *Take Off Your Glasses and See* (Thorsons, 1995).

Lorber, Jakob, *The Healing Power of Sunlight* (Merkur Publishing Company, 1997).

Ott, John, *Health and Light: The Effects of Natural and Artificial Light on Man and Other Living Things* (Ariel Press, 1976).

Ott, John, *My Ivory Cellar* (Chicago: Twentieth-Century Press, 1958; reprinted as *Health and Light*, New York: Pocket Books, 1973).

Rosenthal, Norman, *Winter Blues: Seasonal Affective Disorder—What It Is and How to Conquer It* (Fontana, 1991).

Waterhouse, Debra, *From Tired to Inspired* (Thorsons, 2000).

Zane, Kime, *Sunlight* (Penryn, CA: World Health Publications, 1980).

Resources

Helpful Organizations

The SAD Association (SADA)
PO Box 989
Steyning BN44 3HG, England
Website: www.sada.org.uk
The oldest support organization for SAD.

Jacob Liberman, Inc.
PO Box 2243
Sedona AZ 86339   (800) 81-LIGHT
Website: www.jacobliberman.com
Explores the role of light in healing. Also offers Liberman's books, videos, and other products for sale.

The Dinshah Health Society
100 Dinshah Dr.
Malaga NJ 08328   (856) 692-4686
Website: www.dinshahhealth.org
Dedicated to advancing nonpharmaceutical spectro-chrome therapy.

American Holistic Medicine Association (AHMA)
12101 Menaul Blvd. NE, Suite C
Albuquerque NM 87112   (505) 292-7788
Website: www.holisticmedicine.org
Offers a referral service to help consumers find a holistic-health practitioner.

Outside In (Cambridge) Ltd.
31 Scotland Rd. Estate
Dry Drayton
Cambridge CB3 8AT, England
Tel.:+44 1954 211 955   Fax: +44 1954 211 956
E-mail: info@outsidein.co.uk   Website: www.outsidein.co.uk

Useful Websites

www.holistic-online.com/hol_SAD.htm

www.internethealthlibrary.com

www.mentalhealth.com

www.webmd.com

www.ivillage.com (offers a message board on the topic of SAD)

Light-Therapy Equipment Suppliers

Natural Options
Barb Nelson   (800) 457-2565
Website: www.naturaloptions.com
Sells OTT-Lites, the light-therapy system pioneered by John Ott, as well
as other natural-health products.

Bio-Brite, Inc.
4350 East-West Highway, Suite 401S
Bethesda MD 20814   (800) 621-LITE
Fax: (301) 961-5943   Website: www.biobrite.com
Sells light visors, jet-lag visors, sunrise clocks, lightboxes, and other light-
therapy products.

Floatation Tank Suppliers

http://spas.about.com/cs/floatationtankfl/

Index

T

U

V

W

Y